MENTAL TOUGHNESS ADVICE FROM AN AVERAGE JOE WHO RETIRED RICH

10 Easy Proven Techniques to Develop High Performance Habits and Master the Inner Game of Success

PRESTON HUANG

❀ Created with Vellum

This book is dedicated to all the average Joes and Janes who are seeking something not-so-average.

Contents

Acknowledgments   vii
Introduction   ix

1. Mental Training and Mental Toughness   1
2. What Does Mental Toughness Mean to You?   10
3. Upgrade Your Mindset for Success   23
4. Optimize Your Routine: Creating the Habits that
   Will Help You Achieve Your Goals   34
5. Meditation and Mindfulness   41
6. Visualization   52
7. Interrelationship of Mind and Body   61
8. Positive Self-Talk and Positive Affirmation   69
9. Daily Gratitude   78
10. Rest, Recovery and Stress Management   87
11. Success and Failure. What's Next?   98

Afterword   105
Bibliography   111

Acknowledgments

Biggest thank you goes to my family who believe in an average Joe, like me. Your love and support have been my greatest motivation during the tough times. Thank you for always encouraging my interests and pursuit, regardless of how random and silly they were.

Introduction

Are you struggling to reach your goals? Do you feel like your inner game is not up to par? Well, your mental game and pattern of thinking have a lot to do with what you achieve in life. And to be precise, it is your mental strength and resilience that keep you going even in the face of adversity and ensure that you are not derailed from your path. How you react to the different situations in your life speaks volumes about your character, but if you do not have mental strength, the difficult situations in your life will hinder you from turning your dreams into reality. The lack of willpower and self-doubt can be paralyzing if not dealt with and can affect one or several areas of your life.

In this book, I am going to tell you about the simple yet scientifically proven techniques that will empower you to take your mental game to the next level. Every chapter in this book will provide you with an explanation of the tools, the proven science of why these tools work, and the actionable steps you can take to unleash your inner potential and begin your journey toward your best new self. If you believe that you are capable of achieving MORE—more goals, more dreams, more success, or whatever more you want—then this book is created for you.

I have been interested in mental toughness since I learned of the concept two decades ago. Since then, I have researched, applied, and crafted these techniques to help me and others break through the mental barriers and achieve our unique version of success. These mental training practices have changed my lives and the way I live. They are the same techniques used by several high-profile athletes, fortune 500 CEOs, and prominent figures in various industries (medicine, film, book, etc.) to achieve astounding success. And now, you can learn them at your own pace and reap the benefits. Everything has been explained in a very simplified manner to make it accessible to all.

Though the mental training exercises that you are about to read in this book are simple, developing a powerful mind is not an effortless process. You will need to put in the work and be committed and dedicated. The learning curve may be steeper for some people; however, once you have mastered many of these tools and applied them consistently, you will see what a huge difference a trained mind bring to your life. I can't promise that I will turn you into an Olympic athlete or a fortune 500 CEO after you finish this book, but I can promise that when you have an A1 mental game, the challenges that come your way will be more conquerable. They will become your greatest opportunities for growth. The advice in this book will assist you in aligning your actions and priorities with your goals and beliefs. With each small wins, you will learn to over-come your self-doubt and replace it with the newfound self-acceptance and confidence.

I am grateful that I have learned these techniques early on in life, and I have benefited tremendously from them. Because of these techniques, now I can proudly tell the world that I am a retired Average Joe and a successful one. People thank me for how these mental training techniques have changed and shaped their lives for the better. Our mind is a powerful tool. Train it the right way, and you will be an unstoppable force. But for that to happen, you need to take the steps in the right direction. With this book in hand, you will have the roadmap to guide you on your journey to becoming the person you always wanted to be.

No matter where you are at in your life, you can benefit from a stronger mind. Whether you are struggling, going through a break-up or a divorce, feeling stuck in an unfulfilling career, or just feeling like you are in a funk, the good news is you are capable of changing your life circumstances. The hard truth is you have to take action! You are 100% responsible for the actions you take to improve your situations. There will be factors that are beyond your control, but your response to your circumstances is and will always be within your control.

Ready to get in the driver's seat of your life?

Turn the page.

ONE

Mental Training and Mental Toughness

I f you want to be successful and live a fulfilling life, proper mental training is essential. The commitment to mental toughness is something you will cultivate over the course of this book, but first, let's lay down the basic foundation of these concepts. This chapter will give you an overview of the topics of mental training and mental toughness.

What is Mental Training and Mental Toughness?

Mental training is one of the most prevalent terms used in sport psychology. It is a skill emphasized by coaches in almost every sport to enhance the cognitive thinking abilities of the players. Sports injuries are very common in the career of any sportsperson but recovering from such an injury requires not only a proper treatment but also a dedicated mental strength to get back onto the field. But is mental training applicable only in the case of athletes and not others? The answer is no. The aim of mental training is not only to train athletes but also any person who wish to capitalize on their mental capability. Learning how to train your mind and channel your focus will ultimately help you discover your meaningful pursuits and achieve your ambitions in life.

In 2002, Peter Clough et al. proposed a model of mental toughness, stating that mental toughness is more like a personality trait, comprising of four components: control, confidence, commitment, and challenge (Clough, 2002). Their study demonstrated that the concept of mental toughness goes beyond the domain of sports and can be applied to other areas of life. By conceptualizing mental toughness, they aimed to merge the psychological theories with applied sport psychology, ultimately bringing the research and practice closer to each other.

If you look up the definition of mental toughness, you will find that over the years the term has been defined in various ways. It has been linked to other terms, such as hardiness, grit, and resilience. Despite various attempt to define the term, the core notion of mental toughness remains congruent. Mental toughness is an attribute that enables a person to cope with stress in the face of adversity while remaining committed and determined to achieve a goal.

Here are some of the common characteristics of a mentally tough person:

- **High Emotional Intelligence** – One of the most common qualities of people with a high level of mental toughness is an equally high emotional intelligence. The explanation is quite simple. Understanding your negative emotions enables you to handle them more effectively. When you are in a situation that is testing the level of your mental toughness, your emotional intelligence quotient, commonly referred to as EQ, is also being tested.

- **Ability to keep feelings in check** – When confronting with toxic people, mentally strong people approach the situation in a rational manner. They keep their anger and frustration at bay to avoid adding more gasoline to the fire. They keep their judgement at bay because they appreciate the breadth and depth of humanity. They don't compare themselves to others. Instead, they celebrate other's success as much as their own.

- **Confidence** – Since mental toughness is directly proportional to success, mentally tough people tend to have a sufficient level of self-confidence. They display an inspiring and confident nature which leads them to have the upper hand over most things in life.

- **Know how to embrace failure and move past mistakes** – Mentally tough people know that they cannot reach success without occasionally stumbling on failures. They accept their imperfection and understand that mistakes and failures are natural to the path of success. By viewing each downfall as a steppingstone to their goal, they are better at coping with the adversity and channeling their energy to find innovative ideas for their problems.

- **Say no** – Sometimes saying no is crucial to mental health. Mentally tough people understand their personal limits and boundaries and are not afraid to say no to honour their current commitment. If you are someone who says yes to everything, chances are you will overcommit yourselves and put yourself in unnecessary stress. Knowing when to say 'no' is essential to creating a balanced life, especially when it comes to work and leisure.

- **Embrace change** – Change can be painful, but it is the parent of progress. Mentally tough people are good at adapting. Instead of allowing fear to paralyze them, they keep an open mind, search for the positivity in the change and capitalize on it.

- **Self-care is not selfish** – To be the best version of yourself and give the world the best version of you, you must pay attention to your physical and mental needs. Mentally strong people take time to replenish their mind, body, and spirit because they know they cannot serve from an empty vessel.

Tony Robbins, one of the world's most famous life coach, compared developing mental strength to lifting weights. No one ever starts a workout and gets an amazing physique the next day. Building muscles takes time and consistency. You show up at the gym and do the exercises. When your body adapts to the exercises, you intensify the workout, either by doing more repetitions or increasing more weights. With each additional repetition or weights, your body learns to cope with the stress and become stronger. Similarly, mental training is like "push-up" or "sit-up" for your mind. Your mental skills may naturally develop with life experiences, but to optimize your mind to its fullest potential, this requires deliberate training and a determination to succeed in spite of temporary discomfort.

Why is Developing Mental Toughness Important?

The American Psychological Association's 2011 Stress in America survey revealed that the No. 1 reason for people not being able to make healthier lifestyle choices is due to lack of willpower. Whether it is losing weight, quitting alcohol, breaking a smoke habit, or simply trying not to hit a snooze button, all these require a certain level of self-control. Being able to harness your willpower is crucial in accomplishing your goals. Most psychological scientists define willpower as "the ability to delay gratification, resisting short-term temptations in order to meet long-term goals" (American Psychological Association, 2012).

In 1972, a sociologist named Walter Mischel conducted an experiment to test how young children restrain from instant gratification (Walter Mischel, 1970). The study was famously known as the Marshmallow Experiment. During the study, Mischel presented the children with two choices: 1) the children could have a marshmallow now and enjoy it instantly or 2) if the children could wait for 15 minutes, they would get a second marshmallow. Years later, Mischel tracked some of the children down. Surprisingly, he found that the children who waited for their second marshmallow grew into healthier, happier and more successful adults. They scored higher in the SAT. They have a healthier body mass index, obtain higher educational qualifications, and fare better in many other areas of life.

Mischel's findings were later substantiated by a 32-year study conducted in New Zealand, where a team of international researchers tracked approximately 1,000 New Zealand children. The children were observed and assessed for their self-control and willpower during different activities for over 30 years. The study showed similar findings to Mischel's. After accounting for differences in race, social class, and intelligence, children with higher self-control have higher health and wealth outcomes as an adult (Moffitt, et al., 2011).

The studies mentioned above help us better understand how our capacity to delay gratification possibly contribute to long-term success. But what happens when we resist temptation after temptation? To better understand mental toughness and willpower, we must touch on the concept of willpower depletion. Research has shown that when you are trying to maintain a high level of self-control, your brain consumes more energy.

Constant draining of mental strength to resist recurring temptations can take a mental toll on an individual. Willpower depletion explained why a person often caves in to late-night junk food snacking even though he, she, or they have successfully avoided consuming doughnuts, cookies, and soft drinks in the office all day.

The concept of willpower depletion seems to suggest that we have a limited reservoir of mental energy, but this does not necessarily mean that we are doomed to fail when faced with several temptations. Regular exertion of self-control, in fact, can be beneficial to your willpower strength long term. Referring back to Tony Robbin's analogy of mental strength and weightlifting, weightlifting may exhaust your muscles short-term, but long-term it improves your strength.

Benefits of Mental Training

Mental training is not only beneficial for athletes. It can be valuable to anyone on a day-to-day basis. Your performance at work and your level of satisfaction in life can both be enhanced if you engage in proper mental preparation.

Mental training will prepare you to perform at an optimal level when you are under immense pressure. For athletes, bearing the burden of expectations from fans and coaches can be overwhelming. Imagine walking on to the field, knowing you are representing your school, your state, or your country. Your victory means a win for all the people who are rooting for you. This type of expectation placed on athletes could heighten the level of pressure of the game. This is why implementing effective mental training alongside physical training is crucial for achieving peak performance in the face of immense stress.

In our day-to-day life, we all face several challenges and obstacles. We have all been told countless of times that our success is not determined by the number of times we get knocked down but by the number of times we get back up after our failure. The truth is that not all of us have the will to get back up. For some people, the minute they hit the wall, they turn around and accept their circumstances. For a few others, they rise to the occasion. These are the relentless ones–the ones who refused to accept the self-imposed, limiting beliefs. If Thomas Edison had given up after a hundred failed light bulb, candles would be more of a household necessity than a luxury. If Henry Ford had listened to other people, we might still be looking for a faster horse instead of higher horsepower. Imagine if the jobless, single-mother J.K. Rowling never finished Harry Potter, how less magical the literary world of the 90s children and young adults would be.

Throughout history, we have witnessed many great men and women who overcome unimaginable challenges and reach extraordinary success. They are the people who hit the wall and dust themselves off again and again until they achieve their breakthrough. The fruition of their perseverance inspires and positively impacts the lives of thousands of people. Many successful people attributed their accomplishments to their mental toughness or other synonymous characteristics, such as tenacity, resilience, drive, determination, hardiness, grit, etc. For example, Muhammad Ali, nicknamed "The Greatest" is one of the most celebrated boxers in the 20th century. As a black Muslim living in the United States, Ali faced both racial and religious discrimination; however, he did not let this stop him from attaining greatness. He stated, "Champions aren't made in the gyms. Champions are made from something they have deep inside them-a desire, a dream, a vision. They have to have the skill and the will. But the will must be stronger than the skill."

Myths and Facts on Mental Toughness

Although mental toughness is a term widely used by coaches, sports psychologists, trainers, and business leaders, there are many misconceptions about it among the general public. We have compiled some of the most common myths on mental toughness and explanation to debunk and shed some clarity on the subject.

Myth #1 – You can either be mentally weak or strong.

This is undeniably one of the biggest myths that plagued people's mind about mental toughness. Mental toughness is not an either-or condition. Many people believe that you can either be mentally weak or strong. The truth is there is some degree of mental toughness present in everyone. Mental strength is a spectrum. The more you exercise your mental strength, the higher on the spectrum you rank.

Myth #2 – Mental toughness is only about your mind.

Mental toughness, of course, has a lot to do with your mind, but it does not entirely depend on it. Body and mind are interrelated. There are several factors in life including your physical health that can impact your performance levels. If you are sleep-deprive or feeling hungry, chances are your mind is not thinking clearly.

Myth #3 – Ignoring your emotions is what mental toughness is all about.

Absolutely not! It's quite the opposite. In fact, if you don't pay heed to your emotions, you are essentially not addressing the negative emotions, stemming from certain problematic situation in your life. Mental toughness is about facing your fears and challenges and having the courage to address them.

Myth #4 – You can never fail if you are mentally tough.

Failure is something that everyone faces at one point or another. Even the most mentally tough person experiences failures. After all, no one is perfect. Being mentally tough is about embracing the lessons from failure and staying determined to pursue your goals.

Myth #5 – Mental toughness means having positive thoughts at all times.

Having a positive outlook in life is a part of mental toughness; however, only thinking of happy thoughts all the time is not realistic. Mental toughness is about evaluating your thoughts and the situation for what they are and not allowing your emotions to exaggerate them. For example, if you are having a bad day and another driver cuts you off on the road, you might be drastically more angry toward another driver than if this same situation happens after you win a lottery. Similarly, if you are happy and overly optimistic, you will tend to overestimate yourself and your capabilities. Being mentally strong is about centering your thoughts and emotions so that you can think realistically and act more rationally.

TWO

What Does Mental Toughness Mean to You?

I f you want to train your mind to become mentally tough, you first must uncover what mental toughness means to you. Mental toughness does not necessarily have the same meaning to everyone, but it is important that you figure out your version of mental toughness. For some people, being mentally tough means resisting the endless temptations of indulging in sweets and sugars while trying to lose weight and adopting a healthier lifestyle. For others, being mentally tough means turning down social invites and staying up late working on a passion project while holding a full-time job so that at some point they can quit that job and do what they love. It feels great when we talk about the success stories of perseverance or mental strength, but have you ever thought what it means to be mentally tough in the real world? And, what lies at the core of mental toughness? The keys to mental toughness area clarity and consistency.

High performing athletes know what goals they are trying to achieve and have a plan to achieve them. They also surround themselves with people and environment that support their goals. Even in the world of business, leaders who show a high level of mental toughness have clarity in their vision and determination to succeed. Setbacks may temporarily hinder their plan, but nothing can derail them from their march towards their goal. Though the examples I gave in this book often talk about people with extraordinary success, the truth is success and winning can be as simple as just showing up. Going to the gym even though you don't feel like it. Showing up to work even though you are not super passionate about your job, but that job allows you to invest into your other passion. Consistency is what allows an average Joe, like me, to achieve financial freedom and retired way earlier than the average American.

I think one of the most amazing thing about mental toughness is that it breeds success and it is a skill you can acquire. Mental strength can be built over time if you have the inclination to do so and that is what you are going to learn in this book.

Strategies to Learn What Mental Toughness Is

We have devised three strategies for you to follow so that you can get clarity on your version of mental toughness. Each of these strategies has been explained below:

Define it in your own way – By this, I do not mean that you have to learn any dictionary meaning but to use everyday events to define what mental toughness truly means to you. For example, it can be something like not yelling at your kids when they do the opposite of what you tell them to do, committing yourself to go to the gym an hour every other day for three month, spending at least an hour of quality time with your family on the daily basis, allocating certain amount of time every week to work on your graduate school thesis, etc. No matter what it is, you have to be clear about what you want and write your goal down. Be specific about your goal. For example, don't simply write: 'I want to be fit.' You can be fit in several ways – you can control your diet, you can go to the gym, you can do yoga and so on. You have to be specific in the task that will help you accomplish your goal. Also, decide when and how often you want to perform the task. For instance, I want to lose 10 lbs by doing yoga three times a week for 6 months. Whatever you decide, stick to your plan and be consistent. Action and consistency is how one becomes mentally tough. Saying it or simply writing it down in a diary won't cut it.

Every small win accounts for your mental toughness – This is very much related to the first point that we have just spoken about. Every small achievement or win that you have in life slowly builds your mental toughness. Often you will find people relating mental toughness mostly to the extreme situations and challenges, like the Iron Man Challenge and Navy Seal trainings. Of course, these are the exemplar of mental toughness but is the level of challenge the only deciding factor? No. Extreme situations are definitely meant to test your level of perseverance but you don't have to climb Mount Everest to strengthen your inner game (you totally can if that's what you want). Handling everyday circumstances can also help building mental strength. Suppose you are not a morning person. Then waking up early and getting to work on time will be a struggle for you. By just not pressing the snooze button can be enough of a mental training you need to build a stronger mind. As you can see, there are thousands of little ways in which you can build your mental strength, and these little wins are what will prepare you for the bigger challenges you will face in life.

It is not your motivation that makes up mental toughness but your habits – If you haven't noticed this by now then you should and that is – willpower is not constant. Someday you might be feeling highly motivated while on other days, you might not feel like working at all. The feeling of being motivated is quite fickle. But mental toughness is about building habits that you can do consistently and daily. It is like beating your distractions over and over again. You do not have to be more courageous for that. All you have to be is more consistent. You should not be worried about the obstacles that come your way because that will distract you from focusing on your goals. If you want to strengthen your mindset, you have to build good habits. If you are facing difficulty in cultivating habits, then you should start by building small yet impactful habits that you can do consistently. The habits need not be life-changing ones. They have to be something that you can incorporate into your routine. Don't fret if you deviate from your routine, like missing your workout. Just hop back on your routine and continue doing the task that will help get you back toward your goal. Don't focus too much on the small setbacks. At the end of the day, mental toughness is about what you do consistently over a period of time rather than an instance of failure.

Goal-Setting is a Key Part of Developing Mental Toughness

Life is all about learning to set goals because that is the first technique of building your mental toughness. Goals give life directions. If you do not have goals in life, you might feel directionless and that life has no purpose. Your goal doesn't have to be something grand. It can be simple things that allow you to instigate change within your circle of influence, like cleaning your room. Thinking about your goals help you set priorities and setting milestones will help you progress toward what you want in life. And for that, we are asking you to take a pen and a notebook and write down 10 goals that you want to achieve. As you go further into this book, we urge you to pick one goal from the list and dive deep into developing mental toughness using that goal. Before you write your goal down, we need to learn about a few important things in the context of goal-setting.

You Should Set S.M.A.R.T Goals

Setting random goals is not what we want you to do. There is a particular process of goal-setting that is followed universally by many successful people and these are called S.M.A.R.T goals. The process is aimed at the fact that your goals should be specific, measurable, attainable, relevant and time-bound. If you follow this system, you will have a clear idea of what your goals should look like.

- Your goals should be specific. Specifying your goal means answering the following questions: what do you want to accomplish, when do you want to accomplish it, why is this goal important, who is involved, where will you accomplish this, and which tools do you need? If you say that you want to be more productive then that is not specific enough but if you say that you want to double your business profit in a year by increasing your marketing budget by fifty percent, then that is something very specific and clear.
- Your goal needs to be measurable, so you can track your progress. This can be done with answering the questions like how much? How many? How will I know that I'm on track and when I achieve the goal? Continuing from the previous example of increasing business profit, you can measure your goals by the number of sales, the number of returned products, etc.
- Also, your goals should not be unrealistic. It should be something that is achievable given the constraints you might have. Do research on what it takes to reach your goals. Success don't happen overnight, so plan accordingly.
- Make sure your goal is relevant, meaning it matters to you and aligns with your values. Asking yourself what is

the significance of this goal and why is the goal meaningful to you will help you figure out what goal is relevant and worth your time and effort.

- Lastly, you should put a time limit to attaining your goals. If you do not put a certain deadline, then you can go on for too long trying to achieve something that might not be happening. Also, your deadline should be realistic otherwise it is going to put a negative effect on you by turning the entire process into a race.

Learn the "2 List" Strategy by Warren Buffett

Before you learn what the "2 List" strategy is, you need to know who Warren Buffett is. In case you don't already know him, Warren Buffett is considered to be one of the wealthiest people in the world as he is one of the most successful investors of the 20th century.

The "2 List" strategy devised by Warren Buffet is something that will not only help you focus on your goals but also help you fight procrastination. There are three steps to the strategy:

- First, you have to write down the top 25 goals that you have and you want to achieve.
- After you finish making this list, review it and then circle the top 5 goals among them that you think are the highest priority.

It is important that you finish the first two steps before moving on to the next step.

- Now, you will have two lists in front of you. List A will contain the 5 most important goals in your life to which you will give your undivided attention. List B will contain the remaining 20 goals which you should completely discard until you have completed your top 5 goals.

Once you complete this exercise, you will have mastered the power of elimination through which you can keep aside all of the less important things that may take up your attention, time and energy preventing you from focusing on your most important goals. If you compare your top 5 goals with the remaining 20, you will realize that those 20 goals are nothing but distractions.

Writing Down Your Goals is Important

Now that you know the process of goal-setting and how it should be done, you should understand the importance of writing down your goals and what a great impact it can have on you. There is scientific evidence that proves that the moment you write down your goals, your subconscious self is signaled to start looking for opportunities. Harvard Business Study had found that people who have the habit of writing down their goals are three times more successful than those who don't.

Additionally, there is a bundle of nerves at the brainstem called the Reticular Activating System or RAS that does the work of filtering all the messages that your brain receives and then segregating them on the basis of urgency. Unnecessary messages get filtered out allowing for important messages to get through. This is why you are able to distinguish someone calling your name in the sea of chattering people. When you write your goals down, your RAS is activated and it instantly transfers the message that you have written down is important and that the goal and other things related to the goal should be given attention to moving forward. For instance, when I started writing down the goals for my business, I started to notice more opportunities that help bring my goals into fruition. You may not realize it but it is your RAS that will help you connect with people who are going to be helpful in your journey to realize your goals. Moreover, you become more intentional about fulfilling your goals the moment you write them down.

Design Small Actionable Steps For Each Goal

Everyone wants to achieve something in their life and everyone has goals. Even if you have written your goals down, the problem is that sometimes you might not know where to start. That is why it is essential that you break each of these goals into small actionable steps that will help you to focus on them in a better way. No matter how broad or small your goal is, breaking them into small parts will give you direction and also make them seem more achievable. These steps will act as stepping stones to your success.

For every goal that you have, you can create two or more actionable steps and these steps should be clear and specific. Completing these actionable steps will gradually bring you closer to your goals. Here is a scientific study that proves how actionable steps are important in achieving your goals.

Dr. Gail Matthews of Dominican University had done a research where he divided 267 participants into 5 different groups. All these participants belonged to different organizations, businesses, and networking groups.

- The first group was only asked to think about the goals they plan to fulfill in a four-week period and along with that, they were also asked to rate their goals on the basis of various factors like important, difficulty, motivation and so on.

All groups from 2 to 5 were asked to write these goals down and also rate them on factors that were the same as the first group.

- The third group had an additional task of writing down actionable steps for each of those goals.
- The fourth did not only write the actionable steps along with the goals but also had to share these steps with a friend.
- The fifth group was asked to do the most by sending a weekly report to a friend along with all other steps as mentioned above.

The results of the research showed 76% of the participants who completed the exercise in the fifth group were at least halfway to their goals or had achieved them and this was the maximum percentage out of all study groups.

Your Goals Should Have a Purpose

Your goals and your purpose are not synonymous with each other but to every goal, there must be a purpose. A simple example will help you understand that these two are actually different entities. You might have a purpose in life to be happy but your goal will be to fulfill that purpose by doing something. For example, my purpose is to live a life greater than myself and my goal is to improve people's lives through the service my business provides.

Psychological Explanation of Why Purpose is Important

The experience of a Holocaust survivor back in the days of Nazi concentration camps forms the backbone of the research on human purpose. Victor Frankl, who was a Viennese psychologist, found out through research and observation that when exposed to torture, prisoners who had a sense of purpose were the ones who were able to withstand it.

In terms of psychology, your purpose is the intention of an individual to achieve something that is not only productive but also holds a personal meaning. But you must also understand that every meaningful experience or goal of your life does not make up your purpose. Your purpose is something that is present at the intersection of a focus beyond your self, personal meaningfulness, and goal orientation.

Later on, with the help of several other pieces of research, the observation made by Frankl was proved to be true that the presence of purpose not only lowers the level of stress hormones but also helps in increasing the level of happiness in life.

So Why Have a Life Purpose?

It does not matter how old you are, having a purpose in life is very important to direct your growth in a particular direction. But in order to make it clearer, here are the reasons why we are urging you to figure out your purpose.

Do you want to live your life in the most fulfilling way possible? Probably yes and that is why you have taken up this book. But to achieve anything, you need to have a clear purpose to mark your starting point. The moment you have a purpose, you know whether you are going in the right direction or away fromm where you want to be. You are living in each moment of your life consciously. It is true that having a purpose in life will not simply wipe out all your problems. Obstacles will still come but you will know why you are pursuing what you are pursue and this will give you the mental strength to pull you through the hardship that comes your way.

Purpose gives people clarity. You often hear people advising you to think about the bigger picture. So, what is this bigger picture? It is your life's purpose. When you have that figured out, you will not get caught up in the trivial things of day to day life and you will know exactly what is important to you in the long-term. You will no longer be wasting your time or energy on things that won't add up to your goals. You will be focusing everything on those things that will actually help you to turn your dreams into reality.

As we already told you earlier, purpose gives your life a direction. It gives your life meaning. You will no longer running around directionless but rather have a more intentional approach to life. This doesn't mean that life will be roses and rainbows. There will be thorns and rainstorm. However, you know that you are going towards your goals and that itself keeps you going.

Whenever you are pursuing your purpose, you will feel energized and vitalized. Your purpose is what get you out of bed in the morning. When you have a purpose that you are passionate about, you will not want to go to sleep because you feel like you would rather spend your precious time towards your purpose. But if you are not looking forward to your work and always counting down to holidays, then it is time that you rethink your purpose.

Purpose brings success. Now, this is not something that is guaranteed but think of it this way – if you chase your dreams because you believe in them or because your purpose is properly aligned with them, then you will feel passionate about your work. You will automatically want to spend time doing something related to your work and by giving all this time and dedication, you are bound to get better at it. Keeping all of this in mind, we would say, success is imminent.

It is not motivation that helps you through the difficult times but your purpose. There may be days when you are not feeling motivated but if you have a purpose and you have a 'why', then your unmotivated day will be easier to deal with.

List Your Why's Behind Your Goals

Here is an exercise for all of you that will help you with proper goal-setting and figuring out your purpose.

Remember how we asked you to pick one goal at a time and then proceed with the exercises. So, take that one goal and write all the reasons why you want to do it. These reasons should be something compelling and should make you want to jump out of bed in the mornings.

For example, your goal might be to lose 2 pounds every two weeks. Then your actionable steps should be something like eating more protein and fewer carbs and also exercising at least thrice a week until you reach your weight goal.

Now, you need to list all the things that you will be able to achieve if you accomplish the goal. In this case, it can be things like –

- You will no longer be overweight and can reduce all your health issues.
- You want to be healthy and live longer so that you can spend more time with your kids.
- If you are healthy, you will be able to pursue your passions like hiking or skiing.
- You will feel confident in your own skin.
- People will stop judging you by your weight.

Then, you need to take five more minutes and list all those terrible things that could happen to you in case you do not achieve this goal.

- You will start gaining weight.
- You will have no control over your blood pressure and may even develop other health problems.
- Your overall health will gradually start deteriorating.
- You already have a high heart disease risk in your family and this will increase the chances of it for you.
- Due to your heart disease risks, you might not be able to see your grandkids or even your own kids getting married.

Once you complete this exercise, you will be set for figuring out your purpose and setting goals to achieve fulfil that purpose.

THREE

Upgrade Your Mindset for Success

The way you perceive a certain situation or the way you think can have a direct effect on your actions. So, if you want success in life and gain mental strength, you have to work on improving your mindset and mastering it. Growth mindset is essential in all stages of life and here are some tips for you to develop a growth mindset.

Fixed Mindset vs. Growth Mindset

First, let us give you an overview of what a fixed and growth mindset means. Those who have a fixed mindset have this notion that their talents and abilities cannot change and that they are fixed. They do not really work on improving their talents, because they believe that talents are congenital. They also believe that it is only your talents alone that will help you achieve your goals and you do not require any amount of effort or hard work. These people also pose themselves to the intelligent as they claim to have been born that way. They also fear the fact that if people might look at them as dumb, they will not be able to recover their self-image.

On the other hand, those who have a growth mindset believe that intelligence and learning can both be improved over time if proper effort is made to do so. They realize how their efforts are directly corerelated to their success and thus they know they can achieve more if they put in the work. They believe in the idea that talent can be developed and that you can get smarter if you exercise your brain.

In short, if you want to be successful in life, having a growth mindset is very much essential. When you embrace the fact that things can actually be changed within your sphere of influence and that nothing is static, then you will start making some actual changes in your life. For example, people with a fixed mindset might say 'I am not good at singing' but someone with a growth mindset will say 'Everyone can learn new skills and practice will only make it better.'

How to Create a Growth Mindset?

If you have a fixed mindset but you want to turn it into a growth mindset, then here are some strategies that you can follow:

Embrace Your Weaknesses

In order to grow or change in life, you first have to acknowledge the fact that you have some weaknesses and that is completely fine. No one is entirely perfect and in fact, perfectionism is simply an illusion. Acknowledging our weakness is the first step into embracing it. I used to be very anxious and nervous in a social setting. When I started my business, I had to meet a lot of new people to learn how they run their business. I remembered my palms would start sweating profusely at the thought of having to talk to potential clients or business partners. It was embarrassing. I also would spend hours writing down potential questions and reciting them before going to networking. Thankfully, overtime, this gets easier, and I became more comfortable at talking to new people.

Challenges are Opportunities for You to Step Out of Your Comfort Zone

If you want to develop as a person, then you have to make the best use of the challenges that come your way. The more challenges you accept, the more you will learn. This means that you are agreeing to fight the fear of failure and you are also stepping out of your comfort zone. If you hold on to the excuses to avoid these challenges and remain in your own sweet little cocoon, you will keep missing the opportunities for growth.

You Can Train Your Brain As Much As You Like

The capabilities of your brain are not limited, and it can be trained as much as you are willing to. As we already said before, our brain is like a muscle. It can be reorganized multiple times. Thus, there is always room for growth if you are up for it.

Learning Should be Your First Priority

Your main focus should be learning new things in the course of your life. If you are too focused on never failing then you will lose the potential to develop your mental toughness. You need to prioritize yourself and your growth and not worry about what other people think of you and your failure Also, everyone's path to developing mental strength is different. Don't rush yourself when your progress doesn't seem match others. Think of mental training as a journey and there is no point getting the final destination if you will hate yourself getting there.

Stop Worrying About the End Result

You should not be too anxious or worried about what the end result will be. Who you are becoming in the process is more important than what you achieve at the end. There will be several unexpected lessons that you will get on your journey, and you must have a willingness and openness to learn. If you can develop this mindset, then your end results will also be guaranteed.

Learn to Accept Constructive Criticism

Constructive criticism is a very important tool to learn. If there is room for improvement (which there will always be) and someone is wise enough to point it out to you in a constructive manner, then you should not be offended by it and instead, embrace it with open arms. You should not take any of the criticism personally because that person is simply trying to help. The more you show your resentment the more you will be pushing away those people who genuinely want you to be successful. For this type of mindset, you first need to understand that having a bigger room for improvement does not mean that you have failed. It means that you will have more time to enjoy your journey of mental training and you will reach your goal if you keep giving your effort consistent.

Never Stop Learning

Out of all these strategies, the most important one is that you should never stop learning. You should always be making new goals and figure out new actionable steps to achieve them. Learning is a process, and it never ends. People who master the growth mindset always keep setting new goals after they have achieved the previous ones because this keeps them motivated and focused. Also, do not fret if it is taking you time to learn a few things because it will. This is not a race, and you have to be realistic.

So, are you ready to commit yourself to growing and developing your mindset? If yes, then start applying these tactics in your life today and you will be one step closer to fulfilling your dreams.

As self-help expert Anthony Robbins says –

"All change starts with a decision made in the present moment."

Evaluate Your Core Beliefs

Finding what your core beliefs is an equally important step towards upgrading your mindset. Your core beliefs are those impressions that you carry about yourself and they have a huge impact on your level of confidence and overall happiness. Sometimes self-love and self-belief are not as easy as they sound to be. You will find that there are times when your mind is filled with negative thoughts which can be paralyzing.

There is only so much that you do to change yourself from the outside because there is an entire world inside of you that needs to be dealt with. Every path towards success originated inside you. Your core beliefs are your inner compass. You can practice journaling your thoughts as this is a very effective method for exploring and evaluating your core beliefs.

You need to increase your awareness about monitoring your thinking patterns because they leave a huge impact on your life. They can help build your resilience. But if you are having thoughts that are exaggerated negative versions of reality, for example, "I am good for nothing", then your potential to achieve things in life will become stunted. You need to put an end to your negative thoughts before they go out of control. The best way to do so is to replace them with productive thoughts that can create a positive influence on you.

If you are not sure as to how you are going to identify these negative thoughts then here are some tips for you:

- Do you indulge in too much self-blame? It is definitely crucial that you take responsibility for your actions but it is not right when you keep blaming yourself for everything. Statements like 'I ruined everything' are signals that you are practicing an unhealthy habit of self-blame.
- Do you always focus on the bad news and overlooking the good one? Dwelling over the negative things in life is another sign that you need to work on your thought process. There are people who focus all their energy into the 10% bad events in a day and spend all their time in self-loathing. You need to work on this as well and come with a more positive and realistic outlook.
- Do you keep predicting negative things? If you keep telling yourself that your project is going to be a failure tomorrow, you are instilling that negativity in yourself without any reason whatsoever. If the negative event actually occurs, this would lead to a self-fulfilling prophecy. Self-fulfilling prophecy is like choosing to wear a pair of yellow glasses and saying that the everything in the world is yellow.
- Exaggerating on negative things is another sign that you need to replace your thoughts with positive ones. For instance, you might have stumbled on a question during your interview and concluding that your whole interview is a disaster. This is an exaggeration and not true. The thing about negative thoughts is that it attracts more negative thoughts. If you keep thinking negatively, you will feel increasingly negative.

Replace Your Negative Thoughts

If you are struggling to replace your negative beliefs with positive ones and continuing to have a pessimistic attitude in life, then here are some strategies that you can implement in your life:

Work on One Core Belief at a Time

Identifying your core beliefs and replacing your negative thoughts is a time-consuming process and you should not be rushing it. It is a process of healing and so you should do it one beliefs at a time. You can start the process with the belief that you think is the most persistent of all. But in most cases, you will find that it is not one but multiple core beliefs that actually affect the way you feel or think. But there will also be those core beliefs that are less persistent and usually fluctuate along with your mood.

Understand How the Belief is Going to Impact You

Identifying the belief will not be enough if you do not understand in what ways that core belief impacts you. You can even write down the answer in your journal. The answers will not be the same for every core belief that you have. Some might make you feel anxious while others can intensely affect your level of confidence. For example, if you believe that you do not deserve to be loved. This can impact on your dating life. You may be projecting your insecurities on your partner and be overly and unrealistically selective in choosing your dates because of your insecurities.

Reflect on How Much You Believe In It

Your core beliefs might sound weird most of the times and you might even be laughing at them in your conscious mind. But you have to delve deep into your unconscious level and then see how much impact that belief is having on you. You will also be able to truly reflect on the level to which you believe it to be true. But you need to be truthful and genuine to your own self in order to make this exercise successful. You can rate your belief on a scale of 1 to 10 with 1 being something you strongly agree with and 10 being you strongly disagree with. If you can write all of this down on a piece of paper, then it will bring you even greater clarity in your beliefs. In case you have rated any of the beliefs below 3 and above 8 then you have to go beyond the belief and examine what emotions these beliefs trigger inside of you. For example, if you strongly agree that money is hard to come by, you are likely feeling stress when you spend money. Even when you spend money on something that could help improve your life, like investing your education, you will feel higher level of stress, compared to people who have a positive outlook toward money.

Be Aware of Any Form of Resistance

Sometimes you will find that there is resistance when you are trying to change your old core beliefs. This resistance may not always arise consciously but rather from your unconscious self. The main reason behind this is the fear of uncertainty. You have grown up with your core beliefs and so when it comes to changing them, you might feel the fear of what will happen next. But the moment you become conscious of the feelings that are actually acting to hold you back, you will be able to over-come this resistance.

Disprove Your Core Belief

Now that you are done with the basics about core belief, it is time you take the next step and figure out ways in which you can disprove your core belief. When you disprove it, you will be instilling in yourself how your core belief is not helping you in any positive manner whatsoever and so it is time for it to be changed. You can do this by coming up with three reasons why your core belief is not true. For example, if you believe money is hard to come by, three things can disprove this belief are 1) there are always businesses that are hiring. and can apply for a job to earn money, 2) there have been many people who are in the same position or worse position than yours and they were able to achieve financial success, and 3) Money grows on tree, because they are made of paper. I know the third reason may sound silly but it's affective in disrupting your thinking pattern.

Find Alternatives to Your Old Core Beliefs

When you are have proved to yourself that your old core beliefs are nothing but unrealistic and flawed, it is time for you to find an alternative belief. This one should contradict to your old belief. For example, if your old belief was 'I am stupid', your new belief should be 'I am intelligent' or 'I am intelligent in my own way'. So, the aim is that no matter what alternative you choose, it should be something that you can truly believe in because there is no 'fake it till you make it' in case of your mental health.

Evaluate How the New Core Belief Will Change Your Life

You have to think and explore in what way this new belief is going to change your life. Ask yourself whether you are going to become more confident and happy with this new belief? You can reflect on the answers and jot it down in your journal.

Think About the Consequence of Not Changing Your Old Belief

If you are still skeptical about whether you should change your core belief or not, then I would suggest you remind yourself what the consequences would be in case you don't. This will help keep you focused and not letting you be demotivated. Most people are willing to do more to avoid their fear than for what they love.

Prepare Your Plan of Action

After you have done all of this, you need to prepare your plan of action in order to keep negative thoughts at bay. A plan of action should include things that will reflect on the progress that you have made and ensure that your old beliefs don't pop up.

Uncovering your core beliefs will not be something easy but in the end, it will definitely be rewarding.

The Law of Attraction

Thoughts are very much similar to energy, and they follow the Law of Attraction where they attract similar energy. To put it simply, the Law of Attraction states that whatever it is that you are focusing on is what you will attract into your life. So, if you give your energy and attention to negative things, then you will get back negative things but if you focus on positive things, then you are going to get back positive things in return.

Feelings like happiness, excitement, appreciation, passion, and enthusiasm send out positive energy while those of stress, anxiousness, boredom, anger or sadness give out negative energy. But the universe will not discriminate and give a response to both situations. The only difference will be that you will get back what you give out. So, if you are feeling something, you are requesting the universe to give you more of that same feeling.

So, how can you use the Law of Attraction to your benefit? The simple way is to try and be intentional in your response to every situation in your life. You need to focus on what are the things that you want from your life and then deliberately choose to be and experience those things which make you feel good. Also, you need to believe in what you want. You also need to think of yourself as worthy and deserving of love, fulfillment, and happiness. It will take time but in the end, you will get what you want.

The only limits to the Law of Attraction are your own thoughts. You need to take some time and process everything carefully.

Think about where you are in life currently and where you want to see yourself in a few years' time. You can start by applying the law on small things and then move on to the greater things. You should also keep yourself open to possibilities and practice gratitude. But being successful with this law depends on how patient and persistent you are.

FOUR

Optimize Your Routine: Creating the Habits that Will Help You Achieve Your Goals

Now that you have set your goal to be mentally tough and you have understood the importance of growth mindset in the previous chapter, now it is time that we move on to the topic of why the development of habits is so important for mental strength training. The building of good habits will be the primary focus of this chapter and you will also learn about the science behind good habits. Then, we will move on to how you can build actionable steps that will help you form these good habits.

Neuroscience Behind Habits and Change

If you notice your schedule carefully, then you will see that most of the actions that you perform are all automatic and it is also how your brain chooses to conserve energy in a day. Your habits are what make the person you are and if you are concerned about a particular habit and you want to change it, then you will have to go through the process of rewiring your brain.

Have you ever heard of the term neuroplasticity? Well, it refers to the ability of your brain to adapt to action or behavior that you wire into it. If you do something repeatedly, your brain will form a connection no matter how good or bad the action is. If you act in a particular way today and then repeat the same thing tomorrow, then a specific neuronal pattern in your brain gets triggered and stimulated which, in turn, becomes more reinforced and strengthened in your brain.

A psychologist named Dr. BJ Fogg had repeatedly stressed the importance of tiny actions when it came to the creation of long-term habits. He had said that if you want something to stay then you have to keep doing it repeatedly over time even if it means doing small tasks. But you cannot fail to do them. If you want to write a book but have lost the habit of writing, then start by writing one paragraph each day and gradually, it will become a habit. Your aim is not to do it in higher volumes but to repeat the action consistently. Then, it will become automatic. In order to make it easier, you can start off by doing something that is achievable. There is no magic bullet here. If you want to succeed, you have to learn to embrace the process.

One Tiny Change is What it Takes to Create a Habit

As we were discussing in the previous part, you don't have to be any superhuman to change your habits. All you need to do is make a small change but promise yourself to do is every day. There is a phenomenon, called the Winner Effect, which can hugely affect an individual's success.

During the FIFA World Cup Final of 1994, Brazil had played Italy. It was a truly iconic game since the game was still 0-0 when it proceeded to extra time. To break the tie, the game went into penalty kick, which was when Brazil won by one goal at 3-2. A study was conducted to examine the endocrine system of the fans.

A team of researchers collected samples of the salivary testosterone levels from both the Italian and Brazilian fans. A few minutes after the game, the testosterone and dopamine levels of the Brazilian fans rose high by 50% on an average and 100% increases were also seen. But when the same levels were tested in the Italian fans, they were found to drop by 50%. And all of this effect was because they watched the game. This was termed as the Winner Effect (Bernhardt PC, 1998). There are physical changes in the body of humans and in their endocrine system when they perceive that they have won and quite the opposite occurs when they lose.

Another effect that goes hand in hand with the Winner Effect is the Domino Effect. This effect is based on the working principle of a domino. When one domino tips over the other, there is a gradual increase in momentum. To be precise, each domino tips with a force that is 1.5 times the previous one. Thus, if you think carefully, you will notice the fact that you can literally knock down larger dominoes even after applying the same level of initial force. If you draw an analogy to real life, this example will help you understand how small efforts made with a purpose and direction can help you achieve bigger goals in life, if you keep doing it consistently.

So, if you are trying to achieve big things or be more productive, you first have to start small because even the smallest change counts when it comes to the bigger picture. If you have not performed the same action for a certain period of time, it will not feel natural and thus, it won't become a habit. Coach Margaret Lukens illustrated this with an example saying that she was never a regular flosser and she was never able to make this habit of oral hygiene stick. So, she started to floss one tooth but did it every day. Almost after three weeks of doing it regularly, she felt the need to complete the task and floss them all.

This gradual change seemed natural. She did not even realize when it became a habit.

How to Form Productive Habits by Manipulating Your Environment?

If you want to change your habits and bring in more productive ones, it is not that hard to do. Psychology has proved that your brain will not be willing to spend energy in situations where it does not have to in order to complete the task. But there is also another angle to decision fatigue which says that your brains are more like computers and after a long usage, they are bound to slow down. That is why, when you are tired, your level of cognition is so low.

But one of the ways to prevent this is to stay prepared and guess all the possible sources of friction that might arise when you are trying to do something productive. Once you identify those things, it is your duty to get them done when your motivation level is high. For example, if you want to go to the gym the next morning, keep all your gym essentials packed in a bag so that you do not give yourself any excuse for not going in the morning. There is another benefit to this practice. You will not be squandering away your energy in meaningless tasks. So, if you have already kept your gym essentials in a bag, you do not have to look here and there in the morning and waste your energy. Basically, you will be spending your energy on doing productive work rather than some trivial tasks by simply manipulating your environment.

A simple tweak to your everyday environment can help you significantly in forming productive habits. If you want to get something done, you first have to figure out what is the 'activation energy' that particular task needs. For example, if you want to improve your financial habits and not spend much, then you can choose to leave your credit cards behind when you leave home. You can simply take some budgeted amount of cash and in this way, you will not be spending more than the decided amount. You will be able to overcome the temptations and build your mental toughness levels.

Remember in Chapter 2 when we spoke about the example where the goal was to lose 2 lbs. every two weeks but the actionable step was to consume more protein and fewer carbs and at the same time exercising thrice a week until you reach your ideal weight? But doing all of this, that is, both the exercise and maintaining the diet can make your brain expend a lot of energy which it might not be willing to do. So, in order to make this a habit, you have to work on lowering the activation energy of the task. In order to do that, you can have some fiber-rich vegetables in place of the carbohydrate in your diet and also have some healthy proteins. Continue to do this until you have reduced some weight and then you can start going on a walk or maybe hit the gym. This will make the process easier and something that you can do daily without fail.

You Need 66 Days to Form a New Habit

If you are someone who thinks that you can come up with a new habit in just 21 days then you are mistaken because a time span so short is never enough. The European Journal of Social Psychology had published a study that concluded that a person needs at least 66 days to form a new habit (Phillippa Lally, 2009). The research was conducted by Phillippa Lally and her colleagues from the University College London. The study was performed on 96 people.

One of the most important findings of this research was that even if you miss an opportunity or skip a day during this span of time, it won't affect the habit-forming process that gravely. So, it is safe to say that you can skip a day if you want and yet be successful in forming that new habit.

But you have to understand that the span of 66 days was only an average number. For a person, it might take anything between 18 to 254 days to form a new habit depending on what that habit is. For example, if someone wants to complete 50 sit-ups every day before breakfast then that is going to be something tough and would require a considerable period of time as compared to the habit of drinking a glass of water every day. In the research, there was a sub-group that took longer than the others to form the habit. It is because of this that it can be concluded that perhaps there are some people who are inherently habit-resistant. But you shouldn't be dissuaded from trying just because of this.

The thing that can be learned from this research is that it is not necessary that your habit will be formed in a span of 66 days because it might take you as much as 3 months. And in case of complicated habits, it can be 8 and a half months as well. Give yourself time and do what you are doing consistently and then you will definitely get the desired results.

With this being said, you should stop getting disheartened when you have not formed a habit in 21 days because that is just a myth. You don't have to judge yourself for failing. You need to embrace the long walk that lies ahead of you and you need to stay focused during the length of this journey. The next thing that you have to remember is that you don't have to be perfect. No one is asking you to be perfect. But be consistent. As already stated above, if you make a mistake once or twice in between, it won't be placing any big impacts on your long term success. Give yourself permission to make a few mistakes. What is important is that you learn to build the strategies that will bring you straight back on track even if you have made some mistakes or met failure.

Lastly, you need to embrace the timeline that is required by you to form this habit. Habit building is a process and it does not happen overnight. The society's hype about the 21-days theory of habit formation is what makes matters worse and instills unrealistic expectation in everyone that any habits will be formed by the end of the month. But this does not necessarily have to be true and in fact, it is not true. You have to commit yourself to the system of habit formation and enjoy the process if you want to be successful.

If you understand this theory right in the beginning, then you will be able to handle all your expectations and making these small incremental changes in your routine will become a cake-walk. You will learn that you don't have to pressure yourself into cramping everything in one single moment in order to form a habit.

"We are what we repeatedly do. Excellence, therefore, is not an act but a habit."
– Aristotle

FIVE

Meditation and Mindfulness

N ow, we are going to talk about meditation, breathing techniques and mindfulness technique and how all of this together can contribute to making you mentally tough. A survey showed that 15% of women and 67% of men would choose to get an electric shock over sitting still and alone for even fifteen minutes. This is absurd. Why are we all scared of spending quiet time with ourselves?

What Do Meditation and Mindfulness Mean?

You would often hear elders or basically everyone in your life advising you to put on that tough face even when things go bad. In simpler words, they want you to be mentally tough. When you are pushing through all those obstacles that come your way, life might become too fast for you to settle down your mind and think clearly. If you are not able to think clearly, being mentally tough is not possible. That is why you need to learn the concept of mindfulness.

Have you ever indulged in time-travel (not in reality but in your head)? If yes, then you know what it means to get distracted by your thoughts while your body is doing everything else automatically. If you are aiming to meet your goals but your concentration is not in place, then achieving what you want will become difficult. Mindfulness helps in bridging that gap so that you can focus on what you are doing in your full capacity.

The roots of this particular concept are in Buddhist traditions. Buddhism practice believes in bringing in more consciousness to whatever it is you are doing in the present. If you are brushing your teeth, then the only thing in your mind should be brushing your teeth. If you are answering emails, then your mind shouldn't be wandering off to other places. Mindfulness is the action of keeping your mind where it is and it helps you become more focused. When you give your undivided attention to the task at hand, you are more likely to achieve success than the situation where you let your mind wander off. But if indeed you find your mind going off the tracks, you shouldn't be criticizing yourself for it. Instead, you should immediately bring your mind back to the present situation and focus on the task at hand.

Mindfulness grows with habit. You can do it anytime you like, for example, when you are running, eating, cooking or even spending quality time with your family. The more you do it, the more efficient you will become.

Now, coming to the next most important practice that you need to learn in order to be mentally tough – meditation. Now, meditating doesn't require you to go off into the forest or some utterly secluded place as you imagine it to be. Meditation can be done at the comfort of your own home. There are several scientific reasons backing up the benefits of meditation. It will help you in lowering down your stress levels, enhance your mental functions and also improve your resilient nature. The best thing about this practice is that it is incredibly simple. All you have to do is sit for 5 to 10 minutes and do nothing!

You can do it every morning but whenever you choose to do it, you have to be consistent and do it every day. If you are not a morning person, then choose a time of your own liking and promise yourself that you are going to meditate every day. Sit on a chair or take a cushion and sit on the floor. Make yourself comfortable and close your eyes. In that span of 5 to 10 minutes when you sit calmly, you simply need to focus on your breathing and not anything else. Breathe in and breathe out. Avoid checking the clock from time to time because that will break your concentration. Instead, practice setting a timer.

How Meditation Helps You Become Mentally Tough?

Just like you exercise daily to keep your body healthy, meditation is very similar to that. The only difference is that it is a special form of recovery exercise meant for your brain.

Benefits of Meditation

Here are some of the ways in which meditation helps you:

- You must have noticed how your heart rate increases when you do the cardio workout. Cardio exercises increase your heart rate because it is meant to improve your heart health. So, if a person attends cardio workouts regularly, then their heart will have to work less in order to pump the same amount of blood to every part of their body even when the person is at rest. Our brain works similarly. When you are in the state of meditation, your mind learns ways in which it can enhance its focus and also exercise control over your thoughts. So, when your meditative state ends, even then your power to concentrate and focus remains strong and you attain a greater level of productivity.

- When you do some form of physical exercise, there is a release of endorphins, which are a special form of neurotransmitters. These are the same compounds that are considered to be responsible for 'runner's high'. These same neurotransmitters are also released when you are meditating. But apart from that, some other compounds are also enhanced, and they are GABA, DHEA, melatonin, and serotonin. All of these compounds are responsible for stabilizing your moods, give you a healthy sleep cycle, alleviate depression and also give you high levels of energy. Meditation will also decrease your levels of cortisol, thus, alleviating some health problems like sugar imbalance, bone loss, and chronic stress.

- With every session of meditation, the ability of your brain to focus will increase and become better.

- When you work out regularly, you are able to get a better physique and a relief from the problems of a troubling body image. But with meditation, you get more. Meditation can bring about introspection and self-reflection, which may help you gain insight to your self-image issue. This is because when you meditate, you are able to move past your self-judgment and see the world in a new light. You will be able to build better self-esteem for yourself when you have a positive body image and all of this is possible with regular meditation.

Regions of Brain that Benefit from Meditation

Your brain is composed of various regions and there are some specific regions which benefit from the process of meditation more than the others and they have been explained below.

- Parietal Lobe – The parietal lobe is the part of your brain that is responsible for processing all information that is present in your surroundings. The activity in this part of your brain is found to slow down when you meditate. Humans are social creatures and if you want to feel good, then you also need to be well-connected. The parietal junctures are the regions which are connected to empathy. A 2008 study showed that when people meditated, they showed a greater level of activation in parietal lobe when they heard sounds of suffering from other people because this parietal juncture was exceptionally responsive (Lutz A, 2008).

- Corpus Callosum – The brain has two hemispheres and the corpus callosum is the structure responsible for joining these two hemispheres. According to a study in 2012, people who meditate have stronger corpus callosum than those who don't (Luders E, 2012). Thus, we could say that meditation brings you improved mental health, better focus, enhanced memory, as well as creativity.

- Hippocampus – The NeuroImage Journal has published a study in the year 2008 where they showed how there is a significant growth in the hippocampi when people meditated for a stretch of 8 weeks (Luders E T. A., 2009). Thus, hippocampus is responsible for your mood. Hence, this can help fight depression. The hippocampus is also related to learning and memory. As we age, people often start losing their memories. This research showed that the cortical thickness of the hippocampus improves with regular meditation and this, in turn, can give you a better memory.

There are several other regions of the brain that are benefited from meditation namely the anterior insula (kindness, empathy, and compassion), temporoparietal junction or TPJ (motivation and emotional intelligence), amygdala (fight or flight response and stress) and prefrontal cortex (creativity, intelligence, and brainpower).

Meditation Helps in Building Willpower

We have already discussed willpower in the previous chapters but here, we are going to talk about how you can achieve willpower with meditation. When you want to achieve something in life, there are things that you have to do but you are not really inclined to do. For example, if you are on a diet, you might not be willing to choose salad over pizza but you have to because it is good for you. That is where meditation comes in. It will help you make all these conscious choices. So whether it is overcoming addiction or learning something new, meditation will help you build your willpower to do it and get you started.

Procrastination is one of the biggest barriers when it comes to achieving your goals by doing something regularly. But with meditations, you can enhance your focus and avoid distractions. Every time a thought of procrastination peeps into your mind, you will be able to tell yourself that you are going to do the task today and not tomorrow.

With time, there will be so many temptations that come your way and you will keep having these thoughts of giving in. But whenever you come across such bumps on the road, you need to meditate, and this will give your goals clarity and not let you get derailed.

Why is Mindfulness Essential?

Mindfulness is not only beneficial to those who are involved in the world of sports but even to those outside the sports world. It has been found that mindfulness training, which is especially given to soldiers in the U.S Marines, was able to make the overall well-being of those being deployed to Iraq way better than before (Douglas C. Johnson, 2014). In this training, the soldiers are given the necessary training to stay alert at all times and stay in the moment without giving in to their emotions. This particular exercise was also proven to help them with several complex mental tasks and after the training, they could complete these exercises way faster.

But the key to mastering mindfulness is practicing it daily just like any other workout. In this study, there were 48 marines that were all headed towards Iraq. Before the deployment, there was a mindfulness training class that went on for 8 weeks and there were 31 participants all of whom spend two hours in this class every week. The remaining 17 men were not given any mindfulness training at all. But all men had been given an assignment of mindfulness which they were to perform for half an hour every day. In these exercises, they had to practice focused breathing and also some sessions similar to meditation.

During the ongoing days of the training, several questions were asked to these soldiers. These questions aimed to test their working memory and also recorded their moods. Due to the immense amount of stress involved in the deployment, the working memory of these soldiers decreased. But in the case of the soldiers who were able to perform their mindfulness assignment consistently were the ones in whom the working memory saw a slight increase. A comparison was also made with the soldiers who did not attempt to do their assignment properly and the soldiers who did not go for the training. There were reports of fewer negative moods and an increased number of positive moods in soldiers who practiced mindfulness. So, it was confirmed that mindfulness training can definitely alter the mood of a person. There was no definitive idea as to how mindfulness operates but it was definitely proven that everyone can do well with some mindfulness practice in their life.

In the world of sports, mindfulness has always been treated as a strategy that can help the players perform at their peak levels even when they face a lot of stress. Some of the strategies that are in use in the sports world in relation to mindfulness are as follows:

- The Institute of Sport in England researchers had found out that when players enter the game with the mentality of 'I hope I don't lose' there are high chances of them losing the game very badly (Andrew M. Lane, 2016). It has been observed that such players perform way worse than those who enter the game with the thought 'I'm here to win'. In short, your way of thinking can influence your game to a great deal. Every slight change in your thinking process counts because the more positive you think, it will affect your game directly.
- The way in which the brain of a sportsperson or anyone for that matter responds to stress can be controlled by proper mindfulness techniques. Athletes like Derek Jeter and Kobe Bryant are known to actively incorporate meditation and mindfulness in their schedules. The former coach of the Los Angeles Lakers and the Chicago Bulls, Phil Jackson, had said that he earned the 11 NBA titles as a coach because he taught mindfulness tactics to his players.
- If you visualize yourself succeeding in the match, then your chances of winning increase because you are confident and that mental imagery can have prominent effects on the way you play.
- Players who go through stress and anxiety are often advised to engage in third-person positive self-talk and repeat positive slogans like 'I can do this'. Studies have shown that this helps them to overcome the negative thoughts and focus on what is present in front of them.

Athletes are trained to get into the 'zone' before the game. This 'zone' is their cool-headed state where they can actively concentrate on their game and not on anything else. A world of difference can come to an athlete's performance if he/she is able to maintain this 'zone' despite all the distractions. This is what mental toughness is when they can hold on to this state of mind even when their own self may want to give in for self-preservation.

Meditation for Beginners

There are several styles of meditation and here we want to give you a basic idea of how you can get started with meditation. Each of the different techniques of meditation is linked to different types of mental skills. If you are just a beginner, then you might find it difficult even to imagine that you have to sit for hours doing or thinking nothing. But trust us, it is not that tough and with the help of this guide, you can start right from today. And yes, the easiest way that we have come across is that you should focus on your breathing, and you'll never know when the time passes by.

Concentration Meditation

As the term suggests, this type of meditation is related to focusing all your concentration on a single point. As we stated earlier, this also includes the process where you focus on your breath, or some people even prefer to focus on a single word. You can also try other things, for example, you can light a candle and focus on its flame, or you can also try counting the beads on a mala. In short, do whatever works for you but you have to give your undivided attention to that particular task. As a beginner, you don't have to sit for hours. You can start with 5 minutes and then with time, you can increase your time of meditation to longer durations.

Also, you must check yourself whenever your mind tries to wander off to other places and refocus your attention on that particular task. This will help you work on your power of concentration.

Mindfulness Meditation

This is a technique of meditation in which you simply have to observe your thoughts and let them drift through your mind while you meditate. But the method requires you to not get involved or engaged with these thoughts and simply observe them or be aware of them as they arise and pass by. This meditation aims to help you notice what your thought patterns are. With time, as you practice it more often, you will be able to see how humans tend to judge every situation so quickly and label them as unpleasant or good. You will be able to strike an inner balance with every passing day.

In some cases, people prefer to do a combination of both mindfulness meditation and concentration meditation.

Other Techniques of Meditation

These were only the two most widely implemented techniques of meditation but there are other techniques as well. For example, some Buddhist monks practice meditation by putting all their focus on cultivating compassion. This means they review all the negative events and then present them in a different way in a positive light. They do this by transforming these events through compassion. Some forms of meditation require you to move around and some of them are tai chi, walking meditation and qigong.

Tips for Beginners

If you are feeling overwhelmed with all this information then don't because once you meditate for the first time, you will realize how easy this actually is. So, it is always advisable to start by focusing on your breath and then move on to the complex procedures.

- You should be comfortable with the place where you are meditating otherwise your mind will not be able to relax. Sit still for a few minutes and then simply focus on who you inhale and exhale air through your nostrils.
- You can also focus on things like where you are feeling your breath the most. Is it your chest or your belly?
- Start by focusing on your breath for two minutes and once you get a hang of it, you can work your way up gradually to 5, 10, 15 or even 30 minutes.
- You must be kind to yourself. Even if you find your mind wandering, you shouldn't say harsh words to yourself and all you have to do is simply refocus on the breathing without any self-shaming.

SIX

Visualization

Learning visualization is important. In this chapter, you will learn about the techniques on incorporating visualization into your daily life and how it can benefit you in developing your mental strength.

Let us first give you an overview of what visualization is. You can call it a type of mental rehearsal in which you will think about what you want and then create mental image of your desire. Then, your task will be to do this same exercise daily. For example, you want to be the captain of your football team or a successful entrepreneur. You have to start imagining yourself as one. How would you feel, act, or think if you were already the captain of your football team or a successful entrepreneur? The main idea of visualization is somewhat similar to the Law of Attraction that you learn previously in this book. You will attract what you picture in your mind.

Science Behind Visualization

Have you noticed how you instantly make a memory whenever you try something new? The imprint of the memory becomes stronger the moment you start repeating that task over and over again. The thalamus is the region responsible for this and if you imagine something for long, then the thalamus starts perceiving it as the reality. Your imagination starts feeling more real and something that is attainable.

A study was conducted by the Cleveland Clinic Foundation in Ohio in order to prove that visualization definitely does wonders if practiced in the proper way. They compared people who only visualized themselves working out to those who actually went to the gym. In the end, the results showed that the people who went to the gym experienced a 30% growth in their muscles while those who simply visualized it experienced a 13.5% growth. So, these people did not go to the gym physically but they imagined it and they still got some amount of muscle growth.

Why Is Visualization Important?

Now that you have a basic idea of visualization is, you also need to understand its importance. So, here are a few ways in which visualization proves to be helpful:

- It builds your self-confidence – There have been several studies over the years and all of them have subsequently proved the fact that your brain doesn't really make any differentiation between an imagined event and a real memory. So, if you picture something good, something that you want in your mind every day, your brain will start considering it as something that is real. It will get recorded in your brain just like a real memory. Thus, it can help you in building your self-confidence. Do you know how? Well, when you anticipate that something negative awaits you in the future, that is when you start performing badly due to anxiety. But when you already have a vivid image of your future when you have succeeded, then you get the confidence you need to give your best. All those feelings of insecurity that you were having will vanish into thin air just like that.

- It will increase your ability to focus – Visualization is a process through which your mind is made aware as to what it should focus on and that is also how your perception of reality is made. We have already told you about the RAS in your brain and how it functions as your personal assistant. Visualization enhances the functioning of RAS by noticing all those opportunities that might be beneficial to your goal and then sending them to your brain to focus on.

- You will learn new skills way faster – Another prominent benefit of visualization is that it helps people in acquiring new skills way faster. All you have to do is visualize yourself in a situation where you are actually practicing those skills. Thus, in this way, you are actually stimulating your brain to perform those tasks.

- It will help you override your limiting beliefs – When you perform visualization while you are in a complete relaxed state, it is often called self-hypnosis. Your usual brainwaves are in Beta but when you relax, they move on to Alpha and in some cases, even to Theta. These two are the levels when reprogramming the brain is the easiest. So, if you are on these levels and if you imagine yourself doing something that you had always put off for later because you feared you will fail, then it can have a positive effect on you. But you have to picture the same thing over and over again. This will help you in overriding the previous limiting beliefs that you had about yourself.

How to Visualize as a Beginner?

Visualization is quite easy and so even if you are just a beginner, you should be able to do it without any difficulty at all. Here are some steps that you should follow:

- You need to set or decide what you are going to visualize and once you have done that, it is time for you to close your eyes. Now, you need to mentally repeat the thing that you want to achieve or visualize.
- It can be a situation on which you want to improve in the future. You have to image the situation and the imagery should feel real. This is because the chances of your imagery becoming etched in your memory increases when your visualization looks true.
- Your visualization should emanate strong positive emotions. Strong emotions act like cornerstones of strong visualizations and make them feel real.
- Then you have to repeat the process all over again and keep doing it every day until you start noticing some changes either in your confidence, skills or any other such factor.

The Power of Visualization

Visualization is actively used in several fields because its success is huge. Be it sports or medicine, visualization has been helpful everywhere. Athletes are known to use visualizations techniques in their life for quite a long period of time.

- According to a study, some Stanford male gymnasts who used to rank nationally practiced visualization before performing some complex tricks for the first time and the technique helped them increase their flexibility and also eliminate all the timing errors that they were having previously (Hamada, 1993). Thus, these players were able to increase their focus levels and also reduce anxiety.

- Visualization is applicable to those who have just recovered from a stroke as well. They are advised to picture themselves moving their hands or leg. When these people imagine long and hard about moving their limb, the blood flow to that part of the body automatically increases and the tissue surrounding the affected part of the brain is also saved.

- When youth soccer players were advised to practice visualization, their confidence levels were boosted. They repeated these visions every day and the more they imaged, the clearer their goal became. Eventually, they were able to execute their goals in a better with such an increased level of confidence.

- Visualization has also been linked to comprehension over the ages. When a student is reading something and he/she is urged to visualize it, then their ability to comprehend the meaning automatically boosts up.

A Step-By-Step Approach to Visualization

Since we are discussing the topic of visualization, it is important that you know the story of Roger Bannister. For those who don't know him, he was the first person to run a 4-minute mile and before him, it was considered to be a task that is impossible. But he was the one who shattered this belief. He used mental imagery to do it by envisioning himself breaking this myth. And after that, within a span of two years, 37 people broke it too. But before that, everyone thought it is something unachievable. This is how huge and impactful the power of visualization is.

As already mentioned earlier, visualization helps you to overcome all those self-imposed limitations you have in mind. You need to remember that nothing is truly limited, and the sky is the only limit. If you can immerse yourself into imagining something, then that mental imagery will boost your performance levels by spiking about your self-belief and confidence and you will ultimately get what you wished for.

But in order to make the process simpler, here is a step-by-step list of strategies for you to follow to engage in effective mental imagery training:

- You need to see things from an outside perspective. For example, if you want to see yourself winning a competition, then play the role of a third person and actually see yourself walking up to the stage and receiving the winning trophy. Notice all the details including the look on your face – the determination, the happiness. See yourself carefully. How do you appear? Are you confident? Are you happy? Ask yourself these questions.
- But apart from focusing on all these positive things, you should not forget the negatives as they form an equal part of the process. If you notice any faults in your imagery, then it means that those insecurities are still present deep inside of you. You need to take note of it right in that instance and then you have to reflect on the fact how you are going to react. Keep in mind that your end goal with all of this is that whenever you face a negative thought or emotion in life, you are able to counter it without letting your emotions take the better of you.
- Seeing yourself confident and happy will not be enough. You have to feel what you see. The overall thing has to be a multi-sensory experience. You have to feel the vibe of the roomy you are in and this mind-body connection

will actually help yourself to pull off a smooth
performance.
- You should also write the entire experience in your
  journal and include all the details that you noticed. You
  should also write about what actions you would
  probably take in the face of challenges and
  shortcomings. You can keep this recorded too in case
  you are not the kind of person to write them all down.

Another way in which you can practice visualization is with the
help of pictures. You can create a vision board in which you can
paste all the pictures that best related to what you want in the
future. For example, if you want to buy a car by the end of the
year or maybe a couple of years, then you can paste the picture
of the car you want to buy or past the picture of a house in case
you want to buy a house. If you want to take an African safari
then paste a picture of that from the internet. Whatever it is that
you want, make a collage of all those things on a single board
and keep it somewhere where you can see it daily.

The best practice would be to come with a visual representation
of a goal from each aspect of your life, like, your career, skills,
financial life and so on.

You can also create index cards as they prove to be quite helpful
for some. Take a bunch of index cards and then in each card,
write down one of your goals. Scatter these cards around the
house especially in places where you will access them daily.
Carry them with you when you travel and keep one each in
every bag too. You should look at every card in the stack before
going to bed or before getting up and stare at what you wrote
for a few minutes. Let it sink in. The statements that you write
on the cards should be small affirmations.

You can also practice repeating these affirmations as many times as you want over the course of the day. This will not only reprogram your subconscious but also give you a higher sense of motivation. All those opinions, assumptions and limiting beliefs that you have can be changed with the help of visualization. All the cells in your brain get a particular direction to work on and they put all their energy into it.

If your goal is to lose weight, then you should think about the actionable steps you would take to lose weight and then imagine yourself doing them. It is very similar to playing a video of you in your mind over and over again. You can visualize yourself going for a run every morning, going to the gym or eating healthy. But it should not be boring. Rather you should imagine it all in a vivid and fun manner. You should also surround yourself with the right people, mostly those you admire and want to become like. It is said that your personality is the average of five people you spend your most time with so it is crucial to choose your friend circle wisely.

Although visualization requires you to practice the same mental imagery daily, it doesn't mean that you have to do it all day long. You can pick a fixed time during the day when you will be free to practice visualization daily. You have to strike a balance between living in the moment and thinking about your future.

Warren Buffet has also devised an exercise for those who feel that their friend feels more excited about life than them. The entire exercise treats the stock market as its analogy. You need to think about the people in your life as publicly traded companies. Thus, some of them will do well while others will fall.

So, now, suppose you have only one hour during which you have to select one person from your life who will be in possession of 10% of your life. Then you also have to list the reasons as to why you chose him/her. You have to choose this person based on the fact that you think he/she will keep gaining value in the future just like stocks. Your next step is to choose someone who you think will face a decrease in their value. Then you need to make a list of the qualities of these two people in two separate columns.

When you look at the list of the qualities you listed for the person who will face an increase in value, you will see that those qualities are not inherent and gained over time. Alternatively, for the person you predicted to decrease in value, the qualities of that person would include things that would apply to anyone. This means if those qualities can cause devaluation in that person then it means that it can cause devaluation in you too. So, you need to get rid of those qualities yourself as well.

The ultimate aim of this exercise is that you have to work on removing those qualities from yourself which you think are devaluing in case of others and also inculcate those qualities which are present in people you admire.

SEVEN

Interrelationship of Mind and Body

A s the name of the chapter suggests, here you will learn how your mental toughness is determined by your body language. The best example of this is the gymnasts. Have you ever seen a gymnast performing with a sad face? We bet not because they are asked to put on a smile during their act and be cheerful. This means that even if they had the most disastrous day or a bad practice session, they will still be all energetic and smiling.

How Does Body Language Affect Mental Toughness?

Body language has the ability to influence the way you think because it in itself is a way to communicate. Think of all those years in the past when there was nothing called writing. At that time, it was only body language through which people communicated. The Director of Research and Lead Professor at the NeuroLeadership Institute, Josh Davis, wrote a book in which he emphasized on how your body is important for you to be productive (Davis, 2017).

He said that when you ask computers to work for long hours without any break, it is fine because computers are machines but the human body is not and so you shouldn't be expecting the same thing from them. You have to remember that humans are biological creatures. If you consistently want your body to perform at a certain level of efficiency without taking any breaks whatsoever, then it will be similar to a condition where you are demanding the runner to run at the same speed no matter what the circumstances are.

You will notice, that people often forget the biological factors when they make decisions related to productivity. If you think about it, you will also encounter situations where you went to the meeting without having your snack or maybe replaced a bit of your work time with some form of physical activity so that you can get relief from stress. The research that Davis conducted was based on the theory of embodied cognition. Now you must be wondering what that is. Well, it is a type of phenomenon where it is suggested that when you are structuring your days, your biological needs should be given the upper hand. He had concluded that if a person is able to change how he/she treats their bodies, then a considerable positive effect will come to their way of thinking as well.

Over the years, there have been several studies all of which concluded that your thoughts are hugely affected by your body. There is a concept known as power posing in which it states that your testosterone levels can be affected by the way you sit (Smith KM, 2017). So, if you were thinking that all your assertive behavior and confidence are only the result of your brain functionality then you have to think it over because your hormones and body language have a lot of impacts too.

There was another experiment by a social psychologist at Yale named John Bargh. His experiment showed that when job candidates held a very heavy clipboard that is when they took their role more seriously than when they held a lighter one (Joshua M. Ackerman, 2010). So, in short, productivity is not simply when you tell yourself that you are going to do it. It has a lot to do with your body and the impact of the environment on your body.

Now, most people have this tendency to make being over-worked sound like something cool and happening but it isn't. There is no need to take pride in the fact that you worked over-time. Instead, you should be proud of yourself when you work better in less time. This too requires you to listen to what your body has to say and then respond accordingly. This will ensure that you can identify when your peak performance level in a day is and then structure your day around that span of time.

Some of the strategies that you can use in order to work more productively without being overworked are as follows:

- Exercise daily – When it comes to exercise, people overlook the immediate benefits and often look at what they are going to get in the long-term. But thinking long-term is what makes people keep their exercise schedule after work around 6 or 7 pm whatever suits them. They are used to compartmentalizing their lives. We are not saying that this type of thinking is wrong but according to Davis, if you think in this manner then you will miss out on the several immediate benefits that are associated with exercise. It helps you to stay focused on your present life and also reduces anxiety to a great extent. He said that when you consider the emotional and cognitive benefits, then it is a moderate exercise that will help you more and not the intense workout sessions. Your stress hormone levels will be lowered and you will instantly be able to think with a clearer mind.

- Eat and drink properly – When it comes to your level of focus and productivity, it is food, and especially sugar, that will help you maintain both. There was a study conducted in the year 2012 that showed how the unhealthy diets of employees were the reason why they lost focus in their jobs. You have to think of food like fuel just like a car needs petrol. You need to split your lunch throughout the course of the day so that you are never starving. This will also help you reap the benefits of that meal all throughout the day. You can also eat healthy snacks from time to time. You need to think of food as something that helps to increase your productivity at work and not something that hampers it.

- Use mindfulness techniques – You should mindfulness every day. In the book written by Davis, he uses a very simple yet common example to show how mindfulness can help you. A man was primarily waiting at his desk preparing himself for the meeting. But as he got an email in his box and is tempted to reply the same, he loses the time at hand, and then in the blink of an eye, it is time for the meeting. Now, he didn't get enough time to finish the email. So, he is already frustrated and now he has to enter the meeting unprepared. If you think carefully, you will notice that you must have done something similar at least once or twice in your life as well when you ticked things off your list just to get them over with. So, before going into an autopilot mode, just take a break, think about the situation at hand, and then give your response. The break in between can definitely make a huge change.

Mind-Body Connection

The mind-body connection is the term that is used to define what we have already spoken about in this chapter. It states how all your feelings, thoughts, beliefs and even attitudes are connected to your biological functioning and they can either impact you negatively or positively.

But first, you need to understand the concept of the mind. Some people often confuse the mind with the brain but these two are completely different entities. Your mind is comprised of mental states like emotions, thoughts, beliefs and so on. But the brain, on the other hand, can be called the hardware of your body because it helps you in the realization of these mental states.

Also, mental states need not always be conscious. Sometimes, they are unconscious as well. For example, sometimes you might find yourself reacting to different situations in your life without even realizing that you are reacting to it. And all of these mental states have their respective effects on your body. For example, mental states like anxiety or depression can affect you negatively but those of motivation and joy will affect you positively.

Effect of Body Language on Your Thinking

If you notice a self-confident person and their body language while they simply walk down the road, you will see that their undeniable mental strength can literally be felt from the outside. Now, if you compare that same person with someone who is shy then the first point of difference that you will notice is their posture. It is seen that confident people have straight backs and broad shoulders but a shy person usually crouches and has hanging shoulders. This entire characteristic that we have just explained has a particular term to it and it is called embodiment.

Fritz Strack performed an experiment to study the relationship between emotions and facial expressions (Strack, 1988). He did the study on two groups of people where the first group was asked to keep a pen between their teeth and hold it like that and the second group was asked to take a pen too and put it between their lips. Now on observation, it was seen when the people had the pen between their lips, it looked like they were grim but when they had it between their teeth, it looked as if they were smiling. Then the researched gave every person a comic book and asked them to read it and then enquired how much fun did they find the comic book to be.

The results were astonishing. The people who had the pen between their teeth said that they found the comic book more funny as compared to the ones who had the pen between their lips. Now, do you know what the conclusion of the above experiment is? Fritz said that turning a bad and gloomy day into a merrier one is easy when people put on a fake smile.

There was another experiment which was conducted by Germany's Hannover Medical School (Wollmer, 2012). They wanted to prove that facial expressions can affect depression too. Their belief was that if the patients had a lesser number of frown lines on their face then they will suffer less from depression. So, with the help of Botox injections, the frown lines were smoothened a bit. And the result was that among the patients, 60% experienced s considerable improvement in their mood.

Our intentions are what basically give rise to our facial expressions and not feelings. This was said by the Department of Psychology and Brain Sciences at UC Santa Barbara's associate professor Alan J. Fridlund. Traditionally, people used to think that moods and emotions of people are what largely describe our facial expressions but that is not the case. Our faces are mostly about how or where we want a particular social interaction to go and less about the person itself.

For example, when people cry, people consider it to be the person's portrayal of sadness but it is more than that. It is more like the fact that the person wants some kind of reassurance or emotional comfort from those present in front of him/her.

Similarly, when people are angry, it might be that the person displaying the emotion is frustrated or furious on someone or something but apart from that, the angry face is also used to intimidate or subdue the person present in front.

Act Like You Are Mentally Strong

If you want to feel confident and happy in your life no matter what is happening around you, remember that it is always your choice to do that. People have this notion that it is only when they want to do something or achieve something in life, that is when they have to be confident and motivated prior to the task. They have this type of thought process that makes them think if something is wrong from the beginning then maybe it is not meant to be.

But it won't ever feel like it is right when you are just starting out with something new. As already mentioned before in the previous chapters, your brain has the habit of conserving energy for tasks that it thinks is precious. So, what is the way out of this? It is quite simple. You have to repeat the same mental loops over and over again like a habit until the time that your brain doesn't really have to spend any amount of energy in active thinking. But sometimes all of this will simply feel wrong as if you are lying to your own self.

There are ways in which you can prevent that. One of the easiest ways is to smile. It is not necessary to always feel like smiling but the experiment of holding a pen in between your teeth, which is mentioned in the earlier part of this chapter, shows how smiling itself can improve your mood. If you want to become more social, simply go out and participate in some volunteer work. The theory is that if you want to change what you think about yourself, you should start doing that by changing your behavior.

As the feedback loop works between your brain and your facial muscles, you will start feeling better in no time.

EIGHT

Positive Self-Talk and Positive Affirmation

Y ou need to have an idea of how the process of self-affirmation and self-talk can help you in becoming mentally stronger. Having a positive mindset in life is something that is talked about almost everywhere. And yes, it is important that you always see the glass as half-full rather than half-empty. And self-talk forms a very important part of the entire positive mindset process but before we go into the details, it is crucial that you understand what positive self-talk is and the science behind it.

Self-talk is the endless thoughts that you have in your mind throughout the day. Self-talk is not always positive. If your thoughts are negative, then they are going to affect you negatively but if you engage in positive self-talk, then it can be highly beneficial. The key to effective self-talk is that you should never say anything to yourself that you wouldn't think of saying to someone else either. Positive affirmations are the small positive statements used in a session of self-talk. These affirmations can challenge your unhelpful or negative thoughts eliminating them completely. These affirmations will not only motivate you but also help in boosting your self-esteem.

Science Behind Positive Affirmations

There is no magic behind how these positive affirmations work. There is only science but in order to realize that for yourself, you have to promise that you will practice them regularly. Long-term changes through positive affirmations are possible only if you are consistent with them. Steele had come up with the self-affirmation theory in the year 1988 (M.Steele, 1988). The basis of the theory is that if you tell yourself that you can do it or anything that you believe in a positive light, then your sense of self-integrity will get highly improved.

Now, you must be wondering what self-integrity is. It is related to the concept of self-efficacy, that is, your ability to perceive things and the way you respond to things when you feel that there is a threat to your self-concept. If you want to understand how exactly these positive affirmations work, then you have to know about the key ideas that this theory is based upon.

- With the help of self-affirmation, people follow a narrative where they see themselves as more capable, flexible and moral. This is what their self-identity is made up of. But the self-identity that you should seek to establish should be flexible and should not be too rigid. For example, you should not only be someone's son or husband but acquire different roles as the time and situation demand you to.
- The next point in this theory is that you don't have to be perfect, exceptional or excellent in order to maintain your self-identity. All you have to be is adequate and competent in all those situations which you hold dear.

- And lastly, this theory requires you to act in such a way that it will merit praise and acknowledgment authentically. For example, if you tell yourself that 'I am a punctual person', it is because you reflect values and actions that are consistent with the statement and not because you want to receive the praise.

If you want super scientific proof of the effect of self-affirmations on your brain, then there have been several neuro-scientific researches over the past few years that can provide you so. For example, when you practice self-affirmations, MRI scans have revealed how there is an increase in some of the neural pathways of the brain. To be precise, there is a particular part of the brain called the ventromedial prefrontal cortex and is responsible for the processing of any information related to your self and also positive valuation. This region becomes more active upon practicing self-affirmations and self-talk.

Types of Self-Talk

Now that you know how positive affirmations and self-talk work, it is time that you know that different types. Self-talk can be divided into 4 basic categories which are as follows:

- Instructional
- Relaxing
- Focus
- Motivational

What are the Benefits?

In an overall manner, you know that positive self-talk can help remove all negativity and make you feel positive but if you want to know the detailed benefits of the process, then read on.

There have been several theories over the course of years which suggest how helpful practicing positive self-talk can be and here are some of the examples which show the benefits of self-talk.

- According to Sherman D.K. (2009) and Critcher C.R. (2015), any amount of stress that is bad for your health or can affect it negatively can be reduced if you practice positive self-talk.
- C. Logel, (2012) suggested that when used properly, self-affirmations can help you practice less resistance towards otherwise threatening messages and this includes interventions too.
- Also, Richard Cooke (2014) said that when it comes to interventions, self-affirmation can be used to enhance physical behavior.
- People often neglect the negative health messages. But with the self-affirmations people will try to improve with the intent to bring about a change and this was stated by (Harris, 2010).
- Self-affirmations are also linked with academic qualifications and students have been able to mitigate their GPA decline and this was found by (Kristin Layous, 2017).
- Also, rumination and stress can be reduced by self-affirmation according to (Koole, 1999).

There are several self-benefits to practicing self-affirmations as well. You will become less resistant or defensive when threats come your way. Harris et al., 2007 did a study on smokers that revealed that when it came to controlling their urge to smoke and change their behavior, self-talk and positive affirmations ensured that the smokers reacted less dismissively when they saw the graphic warnings printed on the packet (Harris PR, 2007).

But if you consider the concept in the broader sense of the term, then it is safe to say that when difficulties arise, you become more resilient to them. In short, you become mentally tough to reject those things which you could not before. So, whether it is a feeling of exclusion, social pressure or pretty much anything that is bothering you, it will be helpful if your sense of self-concept is advanced.

Also, with the practice of positive self-affirmations on a regular basis, you will be able to generate an optimistic mindset. People have this inherent tendency to linger on their negative thoughts but with self-affirmation, they are able to reduce their negative thoughts more effectively. So, the key is to replace all these toxic thoughts with positive affirmations which will give you a hopeful narrative in life.

Then, there is another type of affirmation which is termed as the healing affirmations. These are mostly focused on your physical well-being. Louise Hay, who is a very popular speaker and author, is the person responsible for popularizing the concept of healing affirmations. But you shouldn't be thinking that you cannot practice the healing affirmation until and unless you are not sick because it is not so. These practices can heal both emotional and physical pain and thus can be practiced anytime you want.

The psychotherapist of the Open Mind Training Institute, Ronald Alexander, had found out that in order to instill in yourself a positive belief about something, then you have to repeat these affirmations at least three to five times every day. You can also write these affirmations down in a journal or diary and when you have time, practice the same in front of the mirror. But you shouldn't confuse the benefits of self-affirmations with that of depression and anxiety because these are not so.

Importance of Self-Talk for Athletes

Sometimes, athletes tend to delve into a series of 'don't think-ing' where they tell themselves 'don't fail' or 'don't miss the hit'. This is toxic and paralyzing to performance because the words are focusing more on what you should not do rather than what you should do. At the first glance, you might think that this thought process can be helpful but it is not because when you think in this way, you will put all your focus on things that you know, you shouldn't do. According to the author Steven Kotler, your brain cannot handle multiple things at a time. It has a limited amount of energy and you should be careful not to spend that energy on things that you would rather not do. Thus, these thoughts bring to the forefront those things which are to be avoided and filling your limited space in the brain with nega-tive thoughts. Thus, before your game, your brain emulated those negative thoughts and remained filled with those same thoughts causing anxiety.

That is why sportspersons are advised to have their own perfor-mance statements. These statements are short positive phrases that reduced your brain's tendency to indulge in automated negative thinking. These statements have another profound benefit, and that is, all the mental clutter that a person has before a game is reduced. When athletes are not aware of what to think, that is when the mental clutter obstructs their thoughts even more thus leading them to a situation where they lack clear directives.

When you are making these performance statements, be specific. And remember, you should not be using the word 'don't' at all costs.

Self-Talk and Self-Image

Even when there were not many pieces of research on the concept of self-image, there is one thing that was present even then and that is, saying good things to yourself while standing in front of the mirror. This idea of self-talk was previously aimed only at women to improve their self-esteem but now it is advised to everyone. But the main aim of anyone trying to do this should be not using any word that is negative.

There was a study conducted in the Netherlands in the year 2013 to find out how self-image works (Anouk Keizer, 2013). In that study, anorexic women were observed when they walked across doorways. But in the observation, they noticed how the women tend to squeeze themselves out even though there was no need to do so and they would have passed perfectly the way they are. A neuroscientist named Dr. Branch Coslett from the University of Pennsylvania said that this was due to how the brains of these women perceived their body to be. Their internal representation of their body suggested that they won't be able to squeeze through that door.

The body-brain connection was studied even before in the year 1911 by Dr. Gordon Morgan Holmes and Dr. Henry Head both of whom were neurologists (McDonald, 2007). They worked on a different scenario. At that time, big hats with feathers were quite in trend. When women used to wear those hats, they had to duck in order to pass but the astonishing fact was even when they were not wearing the hats, they showed the same behavior. This is because they were still seeing and imagining themselves as wearing the hat in their mental state.

From both the examples mentioned above, it is quite clear that every person has an internal representation of how they look. There is a concept called motor imagery. According to this explanation, the neurological networks of the human brain that are used to actually perform some physical movements and those used to image them are one and the same. So, when a person is imagining the same movement repeatedly, that is when they have the same effect on their brain as they would have in case they performed it physically.

So, self-talk is no longer considered to be a simple booster of confidence and self-esteem but also something that performs the internal remodeling. Although there is a new finding in recent researches that states when people use the word 'I', it tends to stress them out. So, using a third-person perspective or using one's name in place of 'I' is often considered to be helpful. This may be a simple linguistic shift to you but it has an impact on a much greater level.

Positive Affirmation Meditations

You don't always have to repeat positive statements like 'I am beautiful', 'I can give this speech' and so on because you can also combine these positive affirmations with meditation. There are several methods of meditations that can be combined with self-affirmation to get some amazing benefits. You can also practice several breathing techniques that will not only help you to relax but also motivate you to start your day on a positive note.

How to Use Positive Affirmations?

Now, we will move on to the topic of how you can use the concept of positive affirmations in your life. If you want to get results faster and increase your chances, then practicing the act of positive affirmations is the best way to do so. You will experience much more relaxed, an increased level of concentration, better sleep, elimination of the fear of failure, faster and efficient learning and also a marked improvement in your relationships. But in order to reap the benefits, you also have to present these affirmations to your brain in a very particular way and keep in mind to follow some rules which are mentioned below.

Stick to the Present Tense

It is important that you frame your affirmations in the present tense because this will give you the idea that it is already happening. So, instead of saying 'I will be punctual' say 'I am punctual'.

Always Maintain a Positive Outlook

The basic aim of positive affirmations is to uplift your mood and motivation levels so maintaining a positive outlook is of utmost importance. If you use any negative words, you will not realize when your brain takes it into the thinking process affecting the whole outcome. So, steer clear of all negative thoughts.

Keep it Short and Specific

Your affirmations should not be too long statements. It should be a phrase that you can remember easily and it should clearly state your feelings.

Insert Mood Words

Mood words have the tendency to instantly boost the effectiveness of the affirmations on your mind. So, if you want to get yourself boosted for a workout, say 'I am full of energy when I go for workouts.'

Always Anticipate Success

Don't be too harsh on yourself and end up limiting the success that you can achieve. The thoughts can be anything that works for you but they should be anticipating success.

Use Text Reminders and Post-Its

Keep your affirmations on text cards, post-its, text reminders and scatter them everywhere. This will ensure that you get to have a look at them throughout the day.

NINE

Daily Gratitude

You need to understand what gratitude is, how it works and how is it related to the concept of mental toughness. Everyone wants something good from their lie, be it a lavish house, a good job or maybe financial stability. But do you take time out from your busy schedule and be grateful for the things you already have? Most people don't do that. You have to remember that gratitude is a very powerful emotion and can impact you greatly if you practice it daily. Originated from the word 'gratia' which is of Latin origin, gratitude simply refers to thankfulness. When you receive something good and you display a positive emotion with respect to that, the action is termed as gratitude.

How Does Gratitude Work?

Every form of gratitude is somehow related to gratitude. If you notice carefully the feeling you get when you say 'thank you' to someone, you will see how fulfilling and happy it is. It is a feeling of pure encouragement and satisfaction. Gratitude also strengthens every relationship and helps it to sustain in the long term. It also helps people endure all adversities in life and bounce back from every failure with double motivation.

"Gratitude makes sense of our past, brings peace for today, and creates a vision for tomorrow." – Melody Beattie

It Brings You Happiness

According to Gordon, 2012, gratitude strengthens all interpersonal relationships at home or work (Gordon, 2012). There is a multi-dimensional connection between happiness and gratitude. You do not always have to express gratitude to others because you can also express it to yourself. You will see how your overall health improves with these simple acts.

Robert Holden who is a British psychologist and wellness expert did a survey on adult professionals regarding gratitude. Out of the 100 people in the survey, 65 of them chose happiness over health. But they also indicated the importance of both in life. Thus, this study also indicated that unhappiness is definitely the root of several psychopathological problems like anxiety, depression or stress.

Simple practices like complimenting yourself, maintaining a journal to note down your gratitude statements or simply saying thank you to others can make you very happy and content. It has also been seen that couples tend to be in longer and happier relationships when they practice saying thank you to each other.

It improves your health

Your physical and mental well-being is also affected by gratitude. Over the past decades, several researchers and positive psychology experts have been able to establish the fact that there is a strong connection between good health and gratitude.

People who keep and maintain a gratitude journal are the ones who enjoy better quality sleep, experience way lesser stress, are emotionally more aware and are genuinely happy with their life (Seligman, 2005). Energy, vitality, and enthusiasm to give more effort to your work are all directly correlated to gratitude.

It helps in building professional commitment

When workers are more responsible, productive and grateful, they are more efficient. According to Algoe, in order to maintain a proactive action in the workplace, workers should be promoted to show feelings of gratitude so that they can build their interpersonal bonds and also trigger feelings of bonding and closeness (Algoe, 2012).

It is also seen that those employees who have the habit of practicing gratitude are the ones who walk the extra mile to complete projects and volunteer to take more assignments. The same goes for managers who practice gratitude as they have been noticed to maintain a greater level of group cohesiveness and also an enhanced level of productivity at work.

Science Behind Gratitude

Gratitude is not anything new and has been present in the world since ancient times. Its benefits were recognized way back in the Roman culture which is evident from the fact that gratitude was stated to be the mother of human feelings by Cicero.

But gratitude also has a close connection with your brain and its workings. There are studies that show it is the right anterior temporal cortex that is responsible for all feelings related to gratefulness at the brain level (Zahn R., 2008). Later on, it was also stated that there are certain differences in the Central Nervous System at the neurochemical level and these differences are what makes certain people more grateful than others.

People who feel gratitude and express it have been found to have a greater amount of grey matter in their right inferior temporal gyrus.

When people give or receive gratitude, there is a release of serotonin and dopamine and these two neurotransmitters are the major ones related to human emotions. They have the ability to enhance a person's mood within minutes. So, the simple conclusion is, when you practice gratitude, you are promoting the release of these neurotransmitters thus ensuring a positive nature in yourself.

There was a study conducted in 2003 which went by the name of Counting Blessings vs Burdens (Emmons RA, 2003). In this study, the effect gratitude has on the well-being of an individual was being studied. It was concluded that out of the patients studied, 16% of them who maintained a gratitude journal showed a reduction in their symptoms of pain and they were more than willing to cooperate with the authorities in terms of their treatment.

Relation Between Gratitude and Mental Toughness

Now that you have a basic idea of the concept of gratitude, we move on to the topic of how it is related to the mental toughness in humans. In the year 2012, Powell and Garlington made a study on people who went through some kind of traumatic experience (Powell- Garlington, 2014). They concluded that a considerable percentage of people in that group was thankful later on for the experience they got. In 2007, Morris, Finch, and Scott had suggested that people who show distress symptoms after a traumatic experience are way lesser than the people who experience growth (Morris, 2007). And, most people were grateful and showed appreciation towards life which showed than gratitude was the biggest area of change.

People started enjoying the little moments in their life and they felt stronger and were able to form more meaningful relationships. They even welcomed new opportunities with open arms because they had started valuing life more than ever before. Everything starting from a beautiful sunset to a smile on a child's face would make them feel happy and grateful for the life they have. Thus, that feeling of gratitude actually helped them swim through difficult times. But it doesn't mean that the difficulties were replaced by gratitude. It is not that. The difficulties were still there but simultaneously, there was also gratitude. In short, these people started showing an inclination towards growth because of gratitude.

So, no matter how many curveballs life throws at you, be prepared to take them with arms of gratitude because this will give an opportunity to grow and learn new things.

Benefits of Gratitude

In the previous part of this chapter, you have already seen how gratitude can benefit you in terms of your overall health and happiness. But those are not the only benefits of gratitude. Here is a full list of benefits that you can enjoy by practicing gratitude –

Gratitude helps you form new relationships – When you say 'thank you' to other people, it not only reflects your good manners but also opens the door to making new friends. There was a study published in Emotion in the year 2014, which stated that if a person says thank you to someone who is new in their life, they tend to strengthen their bond. Also, when you are saying thank you to someone who simply held the door open for you, it is making new opportunities for you.

It improves your psychological and physical health – When people are grateful, they are more inclined towards taking care of themselves. All your toxic emotions will also get removed whether it is resentment, envy, regret or anything else.

It reduces the feelings of aggression – The University of Kentucky had performed a study in the year 2012 according to which it was found that when people are grateful, they are more prosocial. Participants of this study who had a higher rank on the scale of gratitude were the ones who did not have the tendency to retaliate against others. This feeling was constant even in the face of negative feedback. They had high feelings of empathy and exercised more sensitivity in life. They did not have any or decreased sense of revenge.

It improves self-esteem – The Journal of Applied Sport Psychology published a study in the year 2014 which stated that the self-esteem of athletes got highly improved when they practiced gratitude. And self-esteem, in turn, is an essential component to ensure an optimum level of performance. Social comparisons among people are also reduced to a great extent when people develop the habit of gratitude. Instead of being jealous of others who have more riches or becoming resentful towards someone who achieved greater things, people are able to appreciate the accomplishments of others.

It also helps in sleeping better – The Applied Psychology: Health and Well-Being published a study in the year 2011 where it showed how maintaining a gratitude journal was so helpful in improving sleep. All you need to do spend 15-20 minutes every day before bed and write down statements that signify what you are grateful for. Doing this exercise helped them to sleep longer and also improved the quality of sleep.

It improves mental strength – We have already shown you how gratitude is linked to mental toughness but you must also know about the study published in the Journal of Personality and Social Psychology in the year 2003. It was related to gratitude and the attacks of September 11. Gratitude had a lot to do with resilience. The people who practiced it fostered resilience just by thinking of the fact that they have a lot in life to be thankful for.

Ways to Practice Gratitude

In the previous part, we have mentioned only the major benefits of gratitude but the actual list would be endless. And one of the most important things about gratitude that you need to understand is that it doesn't have to be practiced only during some occasions. You can and you should practice it every day. You do not need anything grand to be grateful for. It can be something as simple as the meal you had and the house you stay in because some people don't even have that much in life. Remember that no matter how much less you think you have there is always someone who doesn't have the things you possess.

So, if you are still unsure about where to start being grateful for, here are some steps that you can follow:

Think of 3 things that you are grateful for

You don't have to make a list of 10 or 20 things. It is okay to start small but it is important that you do it consistently. Think about the small everyday details of your life and start noticing things which were always there but you never thought of them like that. These might be things that you had taken for granted before but are things that you can't do without. You can also turn this into a game and promise to yourself that you are going to notice something new every day. Make the exercise fun and exciting so that you can be motivated to do it.

Practice gratitude journaling

We may have used this term a couple of times before but we never really discussed it in depth. Just like you maintain a journal to note down what happened today, gratitude journaling is about writing down things for which you are grateful for. But you have to make a commitment to yourself that you are going to write in your journal daily. The entire concept of journaling about the things you are grateful for works because as you go along, you will slowly see how your perception of life changes and you will start seeing things in a different light. You might have always been thankful for happing such an amazing mother but the moment you write it down on paper 'I am grateful for an amazing mother in my life' you will feel it in your heart and mind. But you should bring in fresh ideas every day otherwise that feeling of happiness will not remain the same. You need to open your eyes to the things happening around you and you will realize that there is a lot to be happy about. Also, you need to expand your mind and think about everything in your life and not just the things that are right in front of you.

Start your own gratitude rituals

Some people practice gratitude with their own rituals. For example, you can say a prayer of thanks before you eat. This is nothing religious. It is simply a token of thanks for the food you have on your table.

Make your gratitude practice social

One of the greatest determinants of happiness is your relationships with other people in society. So, don't stick to material things only when you are practicing gratitude. Broaden your horizons and practice it for people you are thankful to have in your life. And you can even consider including those people in this practice of yours. Now, you must be wondering how. Well, it is quite simple and not so tough as you think. You can simply write a gratitude letter to a person in your life whom you love or whom you are thankful to have. It can also be someone who has had quite an impact on your growth. Another way in which you can make the practice social is by discussing the things you are grateful for at the dinner table every day. Then, naturally the conversation will go on and you might uncover more things to be grateful about.

Absorb the feeling of gratefulness

When you practice gratitude, you will feel happy, content and genuinely happy. There will also be moments when you will find yourself feeling naturally grateful for something. You need to identify these moments and absorb those amazing feelings. In short, soak it all up.

Make a kind gesture

You can also practice gratitude by returning a favor or simply doing some act of kindness. You don't have to be too mushy to be grateful. Simply giving a compliment or helping your spouse out with the household chores are all acts of kindness. Gratitude expression is about showing your heartfelt appreciation and so you can do it by helping others too, for example, holding the door open for someone to pass.

TEN

Rest, Recovery and Stress Management

Although it might counterintuitive, resting and recharging both physically and mentally are important for developing your mental toughness levels. Now, we are going to talk about how managing stress is important and so is adequate rest in both athletes and everyday people. After all, our brain needs a break too!

Why is Rest and Recovery Important?

The 'tough it out' approach to being mentally strong is toxic and you should know why. This is something people start believing from a young age that they have to keep enduring in order to show that they are tough individuals. You might be having a job where you can go home at 5 pm but does that mean that is where it stopped? No, because in most cases, people, after 5 pm, continue thinking about work, finding solutions to the problems they might face the next day and even talk about work over dinner. In short, they are concerned about work at all times.

Even in the childhood years, the kids are bred with the same misconception about resilience. Parents have the tendency to celebrate and boast that their high school kid was awake till 3 in the morning just to finish the high school project. This is the type of culture we encourage. But should it be that way? The answer is no. You will bring up a resilient child when that child is well-rested. When an overworked and under-slept child is sent to school, he/she does not perform well in studies because they have already exhausted their cognitive skills. That kid also becomes moody and does not behave nicely. Do you think this is what resilience means? These are in fact the opposite of what resilience is. And all these bad habits that they inculcate since childhood only gets magnified when they grow up and join the workforce.

Arianna Huffington, who wrote the book The Sleep Revolution, said that people sacrifice their sleep giving productivity as the excuse. But the irony is that when people compromise and spend more hours at work, in the end, they actually end up losing around 11 productive days in a year which can be equated to $2,280.

Then, what is really the key to resilience? It is working hard but stopping to recharge and recover and then repeating the cycle all over again.

This concept arises from biology. Have you heard about homeostasis? It is the ability of the brain to maintain its well-being by continuously restoring and recharging. A positive neuroscientist from the Texas A&M University by the name of Brent Furl was the one who came up with the term homeostatic value. This particular value is used to signify those actions which have the ability to bring about an equilibrium in your body and also ensure overall wellbeing. If you are overworked, your body becomes out of alignment and a huge amount of resources are simply wasted in the process of bringing back the balance and all of this is done before you even take one step in the forward direction.

In simpler terms, if you work for longer hours, you also have to take rest accordingly otherwise you will face an intense burnout. Now you will also need a greater amount of energy in order to overcome the low arousal level you have currently and this is known as upregulation. This, in turn, increases exhaustion even more. Downtime for the brain will help it to make sense of everything that it has learned in a particular day. If there are any unresolved tensions, then those are calmed down too.

Importance of Rest and Recovery For Athletes

In the case of athletes, a major part of their program is about rest and recovery because this ensures optimal performance. But the process also has another benefit, that is, it gives the human body the time it needs to strength and repair itself. Repair doesn't always have to be physical. Sometimes, it is psychological as well. All the stress that the body of the athlete has accumulated is released. The muscle glycogen is replenished and there is enough time for the repair of the body tissues.

Recover again is of two different types:

- Short-term recovery – This is the most common one and takes only a few hours after a match or workout. The recovery largely depends on how intense the workout was and also includes some low-intensity exercises.
- Long-term recovery – This is more related to the specially design training schedules in an annual athletic program that are specially meant for recovery.

Another very important factor and part of this entire process of rest and recovery is getting enough sleep. The aerobic endurance of most athletes suffers when they are overworked and don't receive proper sleep. In some cases, they might also face changes in the level of their hormones. Some common changes include a decrease in the growth hormone (responsible for tissue repair) and an increase in cortisol which is also called the stress hormone.

What Happens When We Sleep?

Facts state that one-third of the lives of humans are spent sleeping. You can become psychotic if you are sleep-deprived for a long time. But most people are unaware of the things that happen when you are asleep. Plasticity is the ability of the brain to reorganize itself and there are a few pieces of research that relate sleep to the concept of plasticity. But there is no concrete evidence about anything.

In the several types of research that have been conducted on sleep, the conclusion that has come up is that sleep is a brain-focused event. In fact, some evidence has also been found that during sleep, neurons join in a network. When neuron networks were grown in lab dishes, even at that time it showed alternate time periods of activity and inactivity. These periods are held analogous to walking and sleeping. Thus, it is guessed that when neurons start working together, that is when sleep occurs.

Stages of sleep

The University of Chicago conducted research on rats, which showed that they died when they were devoid of sleep for two to three weeks. Obviously, similar research has not been possible on humans. But The Journal of Neuroscience published a study in the year 2014 where it stated healthy people develop schizophrenia-like symptoms and hallucinations when they are sleep-deprived even for 24 hours.

There are two different stages of sleep. One is the non-REM or non-rapid eye movement and the other is the REM or rapid eye movement sleep. Theta and delta waves of the brain are the slow waves, and these are present during non-REM sleep. But when the REM activity is monitored, the electrical state is somewhat like a paralyzed person who is not able to move his muscles even though he is alive.

There is a certain condition called sleep paralysis where people experience odd hallucinations in the middle of the night, for example, a shadow hovering in the room or a hand tightening at their neck, while they are completely lost and unable to make a sound or move. This is basically a sleeping disorder and is quite common and diagnosable. It happens because you woke up before your REM sleep ended.

According to various studies, the brain shows a different type of biology in both these stages. The growth hormone is released by the body at the time of non-REM sleep. Also, some of the brain proteins increase their rate of synthesis and during this protein synthesis, some genes become more active. But all of this protein-producing activity is not noticed in the case of REM sleep.

Sleep Hygiene

Sleep hygiene is everything related to how you sleep and the rituals you do. You may have poor sleep hygiene if you are pulling all-nighters every day and then making up for the lost sleep on weekends. Alternatively, if you are avoiding coffee at night and following a regular schedule for your sleep, then you are practicing good sleep hygiene. Maintaining proper sleep hygiene is essential because it helps in giving you better sleep quality. In fact, people often stress on sleep hygiene as a part of cognitive-behavioral therapy practices used to cure insomnia.

Benefits of Sleep

You already know the importance of sleep but in this section, we want to stress the particular benefits that you can enjoy with proper sleep. There is nothing called making up for lost sleep. It is only a myth because that is not going to help you undo any of the bad effects lack of sleep has brought upon your health .

You can live longer.

You must have heard everyone advising you to sleep for at least seven to eight hours a day and it is true that is the average amount of healthy sleep a person requires. Data was collected from 16 separate studies that were conducted over a span of 25 years. This data was then analyzed by researchers from Italy and the United Kingdom and then the results were published in an article in the year 2010.

The article stated that when a person regular sleeps for less than 5 to 7 hours at night, they were 12% prone to an untimely death. On the other hand, people who have the tendency to sleep more than 8 to 9 hours every night, have a greater percentage of risk towards premature death at 30%.

You can manage your appetite better.

The energy needs of your body are hugely affected by wrong sleeping patterns. In usual cases, your movement is reduced at night and so is the need for calories. But if you continue working and you are sleep-deprived, then you will feel hungry because your brain signals you to do so. This ultimately leads to a gain of weight and bad health.

Children are also gravely affected by sleep deprivation. In a study that was published in the year 2014, it was stated that when children start developing the habit of sleeping less, they get high BMI and also are prone to become obese. As the kids mature, these risks consequently increase.

Your immune system functions properly with optimum sleep.

Cytokines are a particular group of compounds that are released by your immune system when you sleep. These compounds have shown protective behavior for your immune system including their proven benefits towards curbing inflammation during infections.

If you do not sleep, the number of cytokines in your body will reduce considerably and thus chances are that your immune system will no longer be protected. You will have an increased tendency to fall sick. Also, the number of white blood cells and antibodies are reduced with time as you do not sleep for the time required. In a study that was conducted in 2013, it was stated that inflammatory compounds in the body of a human being are considerably increased with the restrictions placed on sleep (Vilma Aho, 2013). These compounds are the same ones that are related to allergies and asthma.

In this research, the study was made on people who were sleep-deprived for around 4 hours every night for 5 days in a row. But before and after this span of 5 nights, the people were induced to two nights in a row of 8-hour sleep. When the subjects were compared to those who have long-term sleep deprivation, it was found that the immune systems of both groups were affected. So, whether it is long-term sleep deprivation or a short-term, your immune system will be affected irrespective of that.

It helps your memory.

Sleep has also been found to help you focus and increase your memory. When people are overworked, they find it difficult to receive information from the outside and process it. They also tend to show symptoms of impaired judgment. Some of them even showed signs of not being able to retrieve any previous information. But if you take seven to eight hours of sleep daily, you can ensure that your brain is going through all the stages necessary. It has been noticed that proper sleep encourages creative thinking, memory processing, long-term memory, and procedural memory.

Lack of proper sleep increases your risk towards diseases.

There are several chronic health conditions that are considered to be associated with a lack of sleep. These are heart diseases, diabetes mellitus, obstructive sleep apnea, and obesity.

Learn These Relaxation Techniques

If you want to combat stress in your day-to-day life then there are some techniques that you need to learn. For some people, relaxation might mean watching Netflix but in reality, it does not really help you much. What you need to do is activate the relaxation response of your body in order to reverse the damage that stress has done to your body. This response slows down your breathing, lowers your heart rate, brings your mind to a balanced state and also lowers your blood pressure.

You do not have to spend so much money on acupressure or a massage because relaxation can be done at home if you know the right techniques. So, here are some to get you started.

Practice Deep Breathing

This is probably one of the easiest methods of relaxation that you can practice. The best thing is that it can be practiced anywhere you want and it relieves you from the stress very quickly. Sometimes people combine deep breathing with some soulful music or aromatherapy.

First, you need to make yourself comfortable and sit somewhere where you will not be disturbed by anyone. Place one hand on your stomach and the other on your chest. You have to take a deep breath through your nose and when you do that, you will notice that the hand on your stomach will rise up. If it doesn't then you are not doing it in the right way. Then, you have to exhale through your mouth and not your nose. You have to try and push out air as much as you can.

If you do it right, then you will feel the contraction of your abdominal muscles. When you exhale, the hand on your stomach will sink in. Continue this process for a few minutes. While you exhale, count slowly.

If you find it difficult to do the process while sitting, you can repeat the same thing while lying down.

Body Scan Meditation

You might have come across this term in Chapter 5 but here you will learn to do it. In this type of meditation, you will be focusing on the different regions of your body. But you will not be relaxing or tensing any of your muscles. You will simply see how you feel.

First, you have to lie down on your back in a relaxed position and your hands should be on your sides relaxed and your legs uncrossed. In the first two minutes, simply focus on the way you breathe. Then you have to shift your focus to your toes on the right foot and simultaneously focus on breathing. You have to feel whether there is any sensation in your foot.

Then you have to shift your focus and you can focus on the sole of your right foot. You have to focus on your breathing too and imagine that the breath is flowing through the toes. Stay in each part of your body for about two minutes. In this way, you can work your way up every part of your body. When you have completed this process of body scanning, you have to sit still and in silence and then notice how you are feeling. You can stretch if necessary.

Progressive Muscle Relaxation

This is basically a two-step process in this one, you have to first tense and then relax different parts of your body in a systematic manner. After a certain point in time, you will realize what tension and relaxation feel like when practiced in different parts of your body. But, in case you had any history of muscle spasms, you should consult your doctor to know whether it can trigger any problems.

Take off your shoes, loosen your clothing and just feel relaxed. Take deep breaths for the first few minutes. Then, start with your right foot and focus your attention on it. Notice how you are feeling. Tense your muscles on the right foot as tightly as possible. Wait in that position till the count of 10.

After that, relax your muscles. You need to focus on how your foot feels as the tension goes away. You need to stay in this state for some time and breathe slowly. Then repeat the same process with different parts of your body.

Visualization

This is another way in which you can practice relaxation and we have already mentioned the different methods in Chapter 6.

Now that you know about all these processes, you can combine all of them into a mental workout that you can incorporate into your daily routine. This will depend on which tools you are planning to use and how much time you have. You should try to do it in the morning right after you wake up and you will have a much productive day ahead or you can also try it at night because it will help you sleep better. But, in case you do not have time in these two periods, you can also do it mid-day.

ELEVEN

Success and Failure. What's Next?

If you think carefully, then life is nothing but a cycle and when you reach a goal, it is not the end. It is only one of the cycles that you have completed. You will always have another one that will begin soon. Sometimes, the goal that you had set before was not right and that is why you didn't feel the joy you expected you would.

What to Do After You Have Achieved Your Goal?

After you have reached the stage you always wanted, you might be wondering what to do and in fact, this is one of the things that most people feel difficult to figure out. So, if you are in the same dilemma, then there are several strategies that you can practice.

- The first and most obvious one is definitely to set a new goal. But this strategy works well in a situation where there is still room for expansion. This strategy is very common among entrepreneurs. Once they complete a goal, they get started on achieving the next big goal. There is always some deal that you can bag and the cycle can go on and on like an endless loop.

- You can also try shifting your current goal further. This is somewhat similar to what we previously mentioned about setting a new goal but the only difference is that you are not setting a new goal but only stretching the present one. If you are someone who had the dream of completing a marathon and now that you have done it, you can set the goal of completing an ultra-marathon.

- You can also try other things. If you have achieved what you wanted, you can now go on and look for things from your childhood that you didn't get time to pursue before. If you always wanted to go on a road trip, why not take your car and go on one of the scenic road trips in the country. Or, you can learn to play guitar if that was something you always wanted.

- You can also take a break. Yes, that is definitely a good idea if your goal was something that was long and has exhausted you, then it would definitely be a great idea to take a break. Simply smell the roses, read a book or spend time with your family.

- You can also join the community of the same niche you were associated with. For example, if you wanted to complete your research on a subject in History and now that you have done it, you can find some historical communities that align with your thoughts and then get a membership. You will still stay in touch with what you are passionate about and you can also help others with your experiences in the matter.

- But the most important thing is to keep going. Don't let your life come to a standstill. That is the most painful thing. Keep going and keep enjoying life in the process. You can change goals or try something new or even quit and spend time with loved ones. But whatever you do, don't isolate yourself or let things crumble after you have achieved a goal.

Reflect On Who You Have Become

When you have completed a journey, you will no longer be the same person you used to be before. When you set a goal and achieve it, you gain experiences and these experiences are what will change you. That is why people say don't focus on what you will get but on the journey because that is your reward.

For example, if your goal was to lose 30 pounds, then after you have achieved it, you will have gained way more than the result. You will have developed a focused and balanced lifestyle by then. You will have a proper diet and you will also have given up junk food. This new and renewed lifestyle is the greatest reward of all. The tangible change in your body is not your ultimate reward but the willpower and discipline you gained throughout the journey are what matters the most.

The same thing will apply to you if you decide to run your own business after quitting the job. There are so many people who dream of doing this but very few people actually have the courage and determination to do it. If you have done it and now you are your own boss, then you know the feeling.

If you look back on your journey, then you will notice that there will be so many changes that might have come to you as a person and changed you for the better. You will see the personal development that you have made in life. It is not always about money or a good body or any such material things. These things will come and go but the experiences you gain will remain with you guiding you throughout your life.

You Can Face Arrival Fallacy

Arrival fallacy is a term used to denote the feeling that sometimes people expect to be happy after reaching the goal but in reality, they aren't as happy as they expected to be. Do you know why this happens? Well, it is mostly because when you finally arrive at your destination, you have the expectation that you are going to reach it and so that particular thought has, over time, already been incorporated in your happiness. Whatever your new state of being is, you have already become adjusted to it. And then there is the feeling of the revelation of another goal as soon as you reach one goal. You know that you have another hill in front of you that you want to climb.

You also realize on reaching a goal that sometimes working towards something that you want to achieve is more joyful and exciting that actually hitting that target. So, what do you gather from all that we have said so far regarding arrival fallacy? The lesson is that you should be happy with your present because, in your present, you have this atmosphere of growth where you are working towards the dream you had always wanted to come true. This entire effect has a term to it and it is known as pre-goal attainment positive effect.

So, there will be times when you will find yourself thinking too much about that goal you have or the happiness you will receive on reaching it. You need to catch yourself in the act and then remind yourself, that you need to enjoy your life as it is in the present. You don't have to think about the happiness that is present for you in the end but rather on the days that you are spending 'now' because this 'now' is the most fun part of your journey.

But the presence of arrival fallacy does not mean you will not receive happiness on pursuing your goals. What we meant to say is that the process, as well as the goal, is important in equal measures.

Success and Fulfillment

Success and fulfillment are two different concepts that you need to understand fully. You might have achieved great successes in life but that doesn't make you fulfilled. Your ultimate failure is when you have achieved success but that didn't give you fulfillment. Most people will tell you the same thing. They believe that fulfillment comes automatically upon reaching a certain point in your career.

What we said above is evident from the amount of depression faced by so many entrepreneurs. Entrepreneurs have this achieving mentality at all times. Whenever they have achieved one goal, they have this habit of pushing their goals further or coming up with a new goal instantly. They simply don't stop this process for the sake of anything. They don't even have the habit of celebrating their successes or acknowledging any of the accomplishments they have made. So, have you really achieved something if you are not happy and fulfilled with your accomplishments? No, right?

But if you think about it carefully, fulfillment is not that difficult to come by. You simply have to do the right thing. It is about contribution, celebration and more importantly, gratitude. And by this, we do not mean that you wait. You have to do all of these things right now. You have to care for yourself because if you don't, no one will. You need to realize how fortunate you really are and this can be felt by a simple act of contribution. The sense of fulfillment usually starts flooding at the moment you shift your way of thinking from that of scarcity to abundance.

Traditionally, success has always been defined in terms of power or money. It is riding that expensive car or buying that dream house or commanding a whole room full of employees. But is that all? No, because all of this will not give you fulfillment. No matter how much power or money you earn over the years, it does not really correlate to your happiness. They are only a part of the bigger picture. We are not saying that they are unimportant because, without them, your picture will be incomplete. But in order to make the picture complete, you also need to feel content and satisfied with what you have.

Afterword

Thank you for making it through to the end of *Mental Toughness Advice From an Average Joe Who Retired Rich: 10 Easy Proven Techniques to Develop High Performance Habits and Master the Inner Game of Success*, let's hope it was informative and able to provide you with a few tools you can use to achieve your goals whatever they may be.

In this book, I have tried to put together a revolutionary method that will help you achieve all that you want in your life be it fulfillment, happiness or success. So, there is no need to fear the elusive challenges that life will put in front of you because with the techniques mentioned in this book, you can conquer anything and everything you want. All the struggles that you face in your life can be overcome if you develop your mental toughness. You need to master the art of self-discovery and believing in your own abilities and that is what I have aimed for in this book.

How many times have you come across situations when you didn't want to do something but had to do it anyway? It should be many because it happens to everyone. Or, do you find yourself making excused to come home early from work or skip your workouts? If yes, then what you lack is willpower and determination to work. Life will throw obstacles in your path but it is your duty to overcome them with the help of various strategies. You have to welcome the challenge with open arms and this can be done if you start working upon increasing your mental toughness.

When it comes to achieving success in life, be it in sports or any other sphere of your life, you need mental toughness because that is what keeps you going even when you don't want to. No matter challenges come your way, you have to persevere and if you follow the techniques mentioned here, fulfilling the challenges and achieving your goal will no longer seem to be impossible. You will be able to build an unrelenting and unbreakable commitment to your goals and aspirations. You will start seeing obstacles for the temporary things that they are and you will no longer fear what is to come.

In this book, I have explained the difference between motivation and commitment. Motivation definitely gets you started but commitment is what keeps you going even in the face of adversity. When someone is mentally tough, they know when and what they want to achieve. There is no ambiguity in their dreams and they are always surefooted. You will be able to make the decisions that are necessary right at that moment. You will not rely on instant gratification to keep you going. You will have your eyes set on your ultimate goal and nothing can make you move. You will realize that setbacks will come and go but you have to get up from them and keep walking on the path that you have laid. You will develop a confident stride and it will emanate from your body language.

I have also spoken about effective goal setting strategies that you should use in order to groom your mental toughness and train your mind in the right way. It should be about creating a clear vision and where you want to see yourself. Set short-term micro-goals and treat them as if they are the stepping stones to your success because they are. You also need to learn acceptance. Every day will bring you something different and you need to be ready to accept it. You should not fight the things life pose in front of you but rather embrace them and learn from them. Mental toughness will help you believe in yourself and give you the feeling that you can handle everything with the same level of efficiency. You will have all your strategies in place to work around even the gravest challenges of life.

Another important lesson that you will get from mental toughness is the ability to focus. As already discussed in this book, strategies like meditation and visualization help you to increase your focus further and take it to the next level. This is a quality that you will need if you want to perform efficiently even under pressure. You will learn how to be consistent. Everything in your life is not under your control, so what is the use of worrying about them? But mental toughness will curb these bouts of anxiety and help you stay focused on the things that are indeed under your control and that will help you succeed. When you focus on the task at hand, reaching your ultimate goal becomes way easier than you might have imagined.

You will learn how to gain back your composure even after you have suffered from a major setback. You will learn methods of quick assessment of the situation that will help you remain unbiased and judge it wise. Then, you will be able to act accordingly. I have also spoken about little acts of gratitude on a daily basis can boost your confidence and feeling of happiness. You will realize that gratitude is that quality that can help you get through some of the toughest moments of your life without even flinching a bit.

Ask yourself what your mission in this life is? Is it to be finan-
cially stable? Or is it to be famous? Or is it something else? No
matter what it is, you definitely want to be happy and reach
your goal. That is why I have created this book to contain the I
information possible that will prepare you for the life that lies
ahead. Something that we have tried to communicate to you in
every chapter is that please do not mistake mental toughness to
being tough on the outside. It is simply not that. No one is
asking you to be a rock-solid person when inside you are shattered. Mental toughness is more about acting according to your
values and not giving up when life gets tough.

You don't have to ignore your emotions in order to be mentally
tough. Your emotions are a part of you and they make up your
character. Instead, you need to understand your emotions and
see what impact they are having on you. Then, you have to
come up with strategies that will not let your emotions cloud
your judgment or control your actions. You don't have to ignore
the physical or emotional pain that you are feeling. You have to
deal with it and then move towards the goal that you have set
for yourself. It is okay to admit that you are not mentally tough
because if you do not acknowledge the fact, you will not be able
to take your step towards success.

In short, mental toughness is just another form of mental health
which ensures that you are mentally strong and that you can
deal with the problems in your life. And mental toughness
should not be labeled as positive thinking because it is way
more than that. All the 10 strategies that I have mentioned in
this book are all a part of mental toughness and without any
one of them, the concept will be incomplete. Once you master
the art of being mentally strong, happiness and success will
follow.

Finally, if you found this book useful in any way, a review on Amazon is always appreciated! As a new, independent author, big-scale marketing is my biggest challenge. I read and appreciate every response. This is my first book and I am very excited to grow from this experience and hopefully write more books in the future.

If you would like to reach out and get in touch with me, please email me at phuang@successcirclehq.com.

Bibliography

Andrew M. Lane1, P. T. (2016). Brief Online Training Enhances Competitive Performance: Findings of the BBC Lab UK Psychological Skills Intervention Study. Frontiers in Psychology.

Anouk Keizer, M. A. (2013). Too Fat to Fit through the Door: First Evidence for Disturbed Body-Scaled Action in Anorexia Nervosa during Locomotion. PLoS ONE.

American Psychological Association. (2012). What you need to know about willpower: The psychological science of self-control. http://www.a-pa.org/helpcenter/willpower

B., A. S. (2012). Find, remind, and bind: The functions of gratitude in everyday relationships. Social and Personality Psychology Compass, 455-469.

Bernhardt PC, D. J. (1998). Physiology & Behavior. University of Utah, Department of Educational Psychology, Salt Lake City.

C. Logel, G. C. (2012). The role of the self in physical health testing the effect of a values-affirmation intervention on weight loss. Psychological Science, 53-55.

Clough, P. J. (2002). Mental Toughness. The Concept and its Management. Solutions in Sport Psychology, 32-45.

Critcher CR, D. D. (2015). Self-Affirmations Provide a Broader Perspective on Self-Threat. Personality and Social Psychology Bulletin, 3-18.

Davis, J. (2017). Two Awesome Hours: Science-Based Strategies to Harness Your Best Time and Get Your Most Important Work Done. HarperOne.

Douglas C. Johnson, N. J.-a. (2014). Modifying Resilience Mechanisms in At-Risk Individuals: A Controlled Study of Mindfulness Training in Marines Preparing for Deployment. American Journal of Psychiatry.

Emmons RA, M. M. (2003). Counting blessings versus burdens: an experimental investigation of gratitude and subjective well-being in daily life. Journal of Personality and Social Psychology, 377-389.

Gordon, A. M. (2012). To have and to hold: Gratitude promotes relationship maintenance in intimate bonds. Journal of Personality and Social Psychology, 257-274.

Hamada, D. R. (1993). Enhancing the Visualization of Gymnasts. American Journal of Clinical Hypnosis, 190-197.

Harris PR, M. K. (2007). Self-affirmation reduces smokers' defensiveness to graphic on-pack cigarette warning labels. Health Psychology, 437-446.

Harris, P. R. (2010). The impact of self-affirmation on health-related cognition and health behaviour: Issues and prospects. Social and Personality Psychology, 439-454.

Joshua M. Ackerman, C. C. (2010). Incidental Haptic Sensations Influence Social Judgments and Decisions. Science, 1712-1715.

Koole, S. L. (1999). The cessation of rumination through self-affirmation. Journal of Personality and Social Psychology, 111-125.

Kristin Layous, E. M.-G. (2017). Feeling left out, but affirmed: Protecting against the negative effects of low belonging in college. Journal of Experimental Social Psychology.

Luders E, P. O. (2012). Bridging the hemispheres in meditation: Thicker callosal regions and enhanced fractional anisotropy (FA) in long-term practitioners. NeuroImage, 181-187.

Luders E, T. A. (2009). The underlying anatomical correlates of long-term meditation: larger hippocampal and frontal volumes of gray matter. NeuroImage, 672-678.

Lutz A, B.-L. J. (2008). Regulation of the Neural Circuitry of Emotion by Compassion Meditation: Effects of Meditative Expertise. PLoS One.

M.Steele, C. (1988). The psychology of self-affirmation: Sustaining the integrity of the self. In C. M.Steele, Advances in experimental social psychology (pp. 261-302). Academic Press.

McDonald, I. (2007). Gordon Holmes lecture: Gordon Holmes and the neurological heritage. Brain, 288-298.

Moffitt, T. E., Arseneault, L., Belsky, D., Dickson, N., Hancox, R. J., Harrington, H., ... Caspi, A. (2011). A gradient of childhood self-control predicts health, wealth, and public safety. Proceedings of the National Academy of Sciences, 108(7), 2693–2698. doi: 10.1073/pnas.1010076108

Morris, L. F. (2007). Coping and Dimensions of Post Traumatic Growth. The Australasian Journal of Disaster and Trauma Studies, 123-129.

Phillippa Lally, C. H. (2009). How are habits formed: Modelling habit formation in the real world. European Journal of social Psychology.

Powell- Garlington, F. (2014). Emergence of discussion of alternative outcomes from exposure to war trauma.

Richard Cooke, H. T. (2014). Self-Affirmation Promotes Physical Activity. Journal of Sport and Exercise Psychology, 217-223.

Seligman, M. P. (2005). Positive Psychology Progress. American Psychologist, 410-421.

Sherman D.K., C. G. (2009). Affirmed yet unaware: exploring the role of awareness in the process of self-affirmation. Journal of Personality and Social Psychology, 745.

Smith KM, A. C. (2017). Winners, losers, and posers: The effect of power poses on testosterone and risk-taking following competition. Hormones and Behavior, 172-181.

Strack, F. M. (1988). Inhibiting and Facilitating Conditions of the Human Smile: A Nonobstrusive Test of the Facial Feedback Hypothesis. Journal of Personality and Social Psychology, 768-777.

Vilma Aho, H. M.-H. (2013). Partial Sleep Restriction Activates Immune Response-Related Gene Expression Pathways: Experimental and Epidemiological Studies in Humans. PLos ONE.

Walter Mischel, E. E. (1970). Attention in Delay of Gratification. Journal of Personality and Social Psychology, 329-337.

Wollmer, M. A.-T. (2012). Facing depression with botulinum toxin: A randomized controlled trial. Journal of Psychiatric Research, 574-581.

Zahn R., M. J. (2008). The neural basis of human social values: evidence from functional mri. Cerebral Cortex, 276-283.

www.ingramcontent.com/pod-product-compliance
Lightning Source LLC
Chambersburg PA
CBHW071013120626
46546CB00003B/1060